"In this honest, probing, and inspiring book, Dr. Matthew H. Bowker sheds light on a life of greater authenticity, bravery, and freedom. *The Power of Being a Subject* will be of interest to anyone yearning to transform legacies of trauma and suffering, escape from unconscious internal and societal forces and self-defeating patterns, and live a more creative and empathic life."

Jeffrey B. Rubin, *PhD, Psychoanalyst, American Institute of Psychoanalysis and Object Relations Institute*

"This is a fascinating study of subjectivity and its relation to one's self. It is also a powerful and moving account of Bowker's own struggle with subjectivity and its impact on both his personal and professional life. An intense and scholarly inquiry into this critical idea and what its pursuit means for our day-to-day lives, Bowker's book is a must read."

James M. Glass, *PhD, Professor Emeritus, University of Maryland, College Park*

"Dr. Bowker's book is perhaps best described as an intimate 'travelogue,' something akin to an innerscape version of Mark Twain's remote journeys. Weaving ideas with personal reflections, Dr. Bowker takes an honest claim to the title of 'poet-philosopher' or 'philosopher-poet.'"

Dan Livney, *PsyD, Psychologist in private practice*

The Power of Being a Subject

Amid countless prescriptive self-help manuals, *The Power of Being a Subject: Transcending Myth and Machine* emerges as a refreshing intellectual cornerstone in contemporary psychology and personal development literature.

Dr. Bowker dismantles the persistent "myth of human mechanics" – the flawed belief that individuals and their psyches "function" like computers or machines. He argues compellingly that authentic self-improvement demands embracing our full subjectivity, with all of its putative dysfunction, and recognizing our agency, creativity, and complexity. Through thoughtful exploration, readers learn how critical thinking, honesty, patience, and bravery can help them achieve deeper maturity and genuine freedom.

This is essential reading for those disillusioned with surface-level solutions and hungry for meaningful transformation.

Matthew H. Bowker, PhD, is the author of more than 20 books and more than 40 papers on psychoanalysis and political theory. He teaches at the State University of New York at Buffalo.

Routledge Focus on Mental Health

Routledge Focus on Mental Health presents short books on current topics, linking in with cutting-edge research and practice.

The Mind of Complex Numbers and the Subject in Analyses
Raul Moncayo

Being a Crisis Chaplain
Delivering Help and Healing in Critical Scenarios
Sidney Dekker and Lance Mergard

A Critical Examination of Irvin D. Yalom's Single Session Consultations
It Is the Relationship That Heals
Windy Dryden

The Power of Being a Subject
Transcending Human Mechanics with Critical Thinking, Honesty, Patience, and Bravery
Matthew H. Bowker

The Knowledge of the Psychoanalyst
Raul Moncayo

Elements of Faith
Psychoanalytic Phenomenon and Lived Experience
Brent Potter

The Power of Being a Subject
Transcending Myth and Machine
Matthew H. Bowker

For more information about this series, please visit: www.routledge.com/Routledge-Focus-on-Mental-Health/book-series/RFMH

The Power of Being a Subject

Transcending Myth and Machine

Matthew H. Bowker

Routledge
Taylor & Francis Group
NEW YORK AND LONDON

First published 2026
by Routledge
605 Third Avenue, New York, NY 10158

and by Routledge
4 Park Square, Milton Park, Abingdon, Oxon, OX14 4RN

Routledge is an imprint of the Taylor & Francis Group, an informa business

ISBN: 978-1-041-04009-5 (hbk)
ISBN: 978-1-041-04012-5 (pbk)
ISBN: 978-1-003-62639-8 (ebk)

DOI: 10.4324/9781003626398

Typeset in Times New Roman
by Apex CoVantage, LLC

For Zoe and Julie

Contents

About the Author

Matthew H. Bowker (M.H. Bowker), PhD, is an internationally recognized scholar and thought leader in psychology and political theory. Educated at Columbia University and the University of Maryland, College Park, he has taught and researched in universities for 25 years. He is currently a research associate professor in the Department of Psychology at SUNY, the University at Buffalo in Buffalo, New York. Dr. Bowker is the author of more than 20 published or forthcoming books, as well as over 40 scholarly articles and chapters spanning diverse fields and genres. He founded and co-edits Routledge's cutting-edge book series, Psychoanalytic Political Theory, and holds several other advisory and editorial positions, such as editor (North America) of the *Journal of Psycho-Social Studies*, associate editor for *Psychoanalysis, Culture & Society*, and editorial board member for several prominent scholarly journals. The U.S. State Department recently awarded Dr. Bowker a Fulbright Specialist grant in twenty-first-century learning, by which he trained faculty and staff at a major university in Singapore in dynamic, subject-centered, and reflexive pedagogies. He has delivered over 50 keynote presentations at national and international conferences and professional development events, on topics ranging from critical thinking to group and organizational dynamics. He has been interviewed on National Public Radio (NPR) and in popular publications such as *The Atlantic* and *Elle Magazine* and elsewhere as an expert at the crossroads of psychology and politics. Some of his recent and forthcoming books include *Walls: Four-Dimensional Essays*; *Getting Lost: Reflections on Psychopolitical Isolation and Withdrawal* (with Amy Buzby, Eds.); *The Destroyed World and the Guilty Self: A Psychoanalytic Study of Culture and Politics* (with David P. Levine); and *Oblation – Essays, Parables, and Paradoxes*.

Part I

Realities and Myths

1 States of Confusion

Looking back, it had been at least six years of serious illness. I was a regular at the local Emergency Room and ended up admitted more often than I would have liked. I had checked myself into a mental hospital four separate times. At home, my nightstand drawer was clogged with pill bottles. I was forced to take a medical leave from work. I had horrifying, extended panic attacks that lasted for days and weeks, alternating with severe depression. When not panicking, I was chronically fatigued.

My psychiatrists amended my official diagnosis to "Treatment-Resistant, Atypical Bipolar Disorder I." If you're curious, "treatment-resistant" really means: *Nobody knows what to do*. "Atypical" means that, instead of euphoric mania, I had episodic, long-lasting panic states that felt a bit like constant near-dying. And "Bipolar Disorder I" is a fairly well-known diagnosis with which some people can function, while others cannot.

I did months of ECT (electro-convulsive therapy), transcranial magnetic stimulation, ketamine infusions, anti-psychotic medication, and more. Nothing helped. My therapist suggested that, instead of bipolar disorder, I had C-PTSD ("Complex (i.e., chronic) Post-Traumatic Stress Disorder") and wanted to treat me for that. My doctor and neurologist argued that I had *Long Covid*, expressing itself in worsening psychiatric complications, severe fatigue, and general unwellness.

Amidst this suffering and confusion, however, I found that I was able to work on my 23rd book, I was well into my third decade of teaching philosophy and psychoanalysis at the university level, I was nearing my 20th anniversary with my beautiful wife, and I was blessed by the love of my wonderful 10-year-old daughter. I had a birthday in May 2024. My family and I went to the beach for a long weekend. In spite of all the things that could have made me miserable, I was content.

In the midst of what some might call "contradictions" – contentment and illness, terror, and happiness – a letter came. My teaching contract at SUNY was to be cancelled due to financial hardship in the Arts and Sciences sector. I would have to look for a staff job at the university or in the corporate world.

DOI: 10.4324/9781003626398-2

The problem was my chronic fatigue meant constant exhaustion. Most mornings, I could only function by dropping my daughter off at school and getting right back in bed, journeying to my classes hours later, expending all of my energy teaching, returning home bone tired, and lying straight down on the couch. Forget the hardship of a new career search: Even if I were successful, I knew I couldn't handle a 9-to-5 job. On top of the lack of fit with my skills and strengths, my body and mind simply weren't strong enough. I would never last.

More importantly, teaching and writing were my *callings*, my vocations. I knew in my heart of hearts that these were the things I was supposed to do with my life. To have to give them up seemed unthinkable. The letter should have been the death knell. I should have been despondent. To my surprise, I was calm.

§

This book is not intended to be a tale of stoic strength. It is not about handling difficulty with grit or tenacity. It is not the story of overcoming obstacles by transforming bad situations into profits. It does not promise a way to get rid of depression, trauma, long Covid, or panic attacks. I have read *a lot* of those books over the years. You may have too.

This book is concerned with exploring the special moments when the pain and difficulty I was experiencing seemed to recede, as it were, into the background. It is concerned with explaining *how* and *why* obstacles softened, when the bad things just weren't so bad any longer, when even life-threatening panic felt survivable. In life, I have come to believe, this is what we need; often, it is the best we can hope for.

These moments of relief had become more frequent and more real for me, so much so that the letter terminating my employment, like other things, no longer felt so frightening. It could be withstood because, while it was deeply attached to my employment and my identity as a professor, I was even more deeply attached to my self and my *being*.

I suppose I hadn't realized how free I had become. I hadn't connected my journey toward subjectivity with a unique and real way for me to *be* in the world. I felt not just surprised, but confused, perplexed by my own reactions.

Why was I not freaking out? Shouldn't I be freaking out? How could I remain calm, even in the face of panic, which is, if nothing else, the opposite of calmness? Why wasn't I more devastated by this blow to my vocation? Why wasn't I more despondent over the state of my mental and physical health, over the poor quality of my days?

§

Before I go any further, I have the urge to say that these were real, honest questions. Put another way, I have the urge to say: *I don't know anything.* I think the urge comes from a humble place, knowing that anything I might say on the topic of being subjective, powerful, critical, or brave should be balanced with a recognition that at times I have been very much the opposite: nonsubjective, powerless, uncritical, and meek.

But, on the whole, it's not true: *I know a few things*. Part of what I know is the result of decades of study, teaching, research, and writing on philosophy and psychoanalysis. When not doing that, I've spent a healthy (I hope!) amount of time reflecting on myself, life, and the world.

So, perhaps I should say: *I don't know anything you don't know*. This helps me to feel that there is something manifestly discoverable in what I am about to write, something that anyone so inclined might find out for themselves. Still, I'm not sure about it: It really depends on what *you* know.

Here's the simple truth: *I can tell you some things I know, but these will not be final answers in themselves. They are more like frameworks and examples that might stimulate some thought or facilitate some development on your part. They have to do with coming alive as a subjective creature.*

You might wonder why I am being so cagey about all of this.

For one thing, I find most self-help books and programs disappointing. A lot of them set up a "guru" model in which people are instructed to ingest a lot of sage advice on "how to live" and "what to do." For the most part – whether because the guru is false or because ingesting a slew of direct advice is not the deepest kind of learning to which we can aspire – these programs don't often yield profound change or lasting results.

For another thing, many (but not all) self-help programs – including the pervasive *ad hoc* self-help advice distributed through popular social media channels – that tell us "how to live" and "what to do" are ultimately guided by the assumption that the goal is to *function better*.[1] No matter the precise message – to "find your purpose," "grind harder," "work smarter," "commit to your path," "release negative beliefs," or even "stop thinking so much" – the aim is to help people find their place in what I call "the great machinery" of family, culture, economy, and society, and sometimes to become even bigger, brighter cogs in that machinery.

Because he is my favorite poet, when I think about "how to live" and "what to do," I think of Wallace Stevens' poem of precisely that title.[2] In "How to Live. What to Do," two people climb a massive rock, perhaps a mountain, whose "ridges" are "thrown / Like giant arms around the clouds." There is no voice up there telling them "how to live" or "what to do." There is no "crested image, / No chorister, nor priest." There is just the sound of the cold wind, blowing with fuller force because they have, momentarily, left behind the "muck of the land" and machinery of the world below.

That sound of cold wind is better than any choir. It is "[j]oyous and jubilant and sure" because the couple has stepped outside of life for the briefest of moments. They have ascended to a special part of the world, a *rarified landscape*, let us say. I suppose that is part of what I hope to share with the reader of this book: the possibility of making contact with a rarified landscape that, in fact, cannot be inhabited *all the time* – because we are regularly cast back into the muck and machinery of life, and because we probably wouldn't want it any other way – but that needs to be accessed sometimes in order to make life livable as a subject. Stevens' poem about finding solace and inspiration from the rock's great height is about finding a way to become a subject and not an object of experience.

If this seems a bit macho, romantic, or gallant, you will have to trust that that is not my intention. As I hope you will see, this book is ultimately about finding a way to catch hold of one's self and one's life. Whether that is to be done by ascending to some metaphorical height or, rather, laterally or obliquely, from the side, or, even, subversively, from below, I leave to your imagination. The point is merely that it is necessary to achieve a critical perspective on the muck and machinery long enough to think about it and about ourselves – even if all we gain is the means to re-enter the same muck and machinery with a renewed sense of clarity, serenity, and power. As I have said, this book is about developing a *subjective state*, which, I will try to show, is the only way to break free from the myths embedded deeply in our psyches, lives, and cultures: the myths that drive the muck and machinery. It is the only way truly to know oneself. And it is the only way to become the author of one's own life.

If developing our subjective capacities means stepping out of the world for a moment, *coming alive as a subject* means turning inward and connecting with something at the very core of ourselves: our *being*. It means contacting that *being* in order to live as what the psychoanalyst Heinz Kohut called a "center of initiative," an agent, an architect, a maker.[3] Developing our subjectivities involves a considerable transformation, perhaps the only one that really counts in human life. It means shedding old skins and becoming new, complex, intuitive, sensitive, inventive creatures, not defined by prescribed paths, goals, or schedules.

Becoming a subject is a bit like dropping an anchor yet still being able to move freely, even swiftly. Subjects feel grounded in something profound, which is their true *being*, yet this connection affords them a feeling of freedom to do almost anything, to go almost anywhere. Sometimes, our own subjectivity may even sneak up on us, leaving us with a bewildering sense of liberty or peace amidst situations where we thought we'd feel differently. My subjectivity surprises me at times, leaving me in temporary states of confusion.

§

Somewhere along my way – and I honestly don't know the place or time – I began to feel that I was *coming alive* as a subject more often, particularly when I wanted or needed to. Again, we are not going to come alive as subjects *all of the time*. There are times in life when, for instance, we must perform mundane tasks like going to the grocery store, taking out the trash, or filling out forms. In these times, we may behave rather robotically, responding to circumstances, only half-aware of what we are doing. This is to inhabit what might be called an objective state.

The real question is whether we can occupy a subjective state when desired or needed. When we need to, can we find that certain strength? There is what I call a "dilemma of activation" here, where we have to ask ourselves *how to know* when it is time to shift toward a subjective stance. I will deal with this matter in Chapter 11, when discussing critical thinking.

Don't worry: Once we learn to see past the confusion that goes along with being subjects in an objective world, things become clearer. Nevertheless, I want to give fair warning: Coming alive as a subject doesn't yield the kinds of outcomes that drive some people to reach for self-help books. Developing my own subjectivity didn't make my physical health better, didn't get me off psychiatric medication, didn't make my marriage perfect, didn't eliminate all my body fat, and didn't land me a dream job.

What it did was to remind me that those things mattered less, in some very important sense, than remaining in contact with the subjective self I had become. While some readers (and some philosophers whom I address immediately below) may worry that all I have said thus far is aloof, selfish, or, by definition, out of touch with reality, keeping our subjective selves alive is the greatest gift we have to offer ourselves and others, our loved ones, our colleagues, our friends, and the world. If subjectivity seems to require stepping out of the world for a moment, to gather ourselves, as it were, it is also the fullest and richest way to be ourselves, to live in the world.

§

Please allow me to say a very quick word about the idea subjectivity, as it is used differently in different (yet, sometimes overlapping) philosophical, political, and psychological contexts. It is my belief that subjectivity is something that we ought to want. Some of us do. Some of us sabotage our own subjectivity, but that is a conversation for a different time.[4] I believe it to be scandalous that we don't teach or facilitate subjectivity – by which I mean that we do not take it as a primary "learning objective" – in pre- and post-secondary schools and in higher education.

Parents want – and if they don't, they *should* want – their children to grow up to be self-attuned, resilient, mature, free-thinking persons, capable of creativity, critical thinking, intellectual humility, and genuine empathy. Teachers and professors want the same – or should want the same – for their students. Therapists and social workers want the same – or should want the same – for their clients. Friends and family members want the same – or should want the same – for their loved ones. And, perhaps most importantly, we want subjectivity – or should want subjectivity – for ourselves.

There are, however, a few detractors of subjectivity whom I will discuss now. In philosophical, Marxist, feminist, postmodern, and critical-psychoanalytic circles, the idea of subjectivity has suffered some criticism of late. I cannot, for sake of space, review the entire history of these criticisms here. They include the work of some very famous thinkers: Martin Heidegger, Michel Foucault, Judith Butler, and more. In each case, however, if you examine the critique closely, you will find that some aspect of subjectivity has been exaggerated while other aspects have been left out. If the philosopher Maurice Merleau-Ponty challenged the notion of the *isolated* subject with a *detached* mind, others have worried about the subject as *essentialist*, *self-sovereign*, or *colonial*.[5]

In what will seem to philosophers to be an all-too-brief statement, let me try to set aside these concerns for now. These versions of subjectivity, with their exaggerated features and out-sized aspects of the subject, do not reflect what I mean by subjectivity and do not really refer to the subject discussed in my work. The subjects I am concerned with are not essentializing, self-sovereign colonialists. Well, I suppose they *could be*, but those qualities have to do with personal and cultural problems arising beside the issue of their maturation into healthy subjects.

The subject and the subjectivity I speak of are a state of selfhood, a coherent personality, a person. To achieve this state requires authenticity and coherent self-boundaries as much as it engenders humility before and empathy for (and even the capacity to feel guilty for harming) other subjects and would-be subjects. Rather than following the trend set by the thinkers named above, attacking the subject and its capacity to think and act with a degree of freedom and autonomy, I have written extensively in defense of the healthy subjectivity that is necessary for psychological maturity and self-flourishing. If the reader is interested, there are a few works to which I can refer you where this position is more fully explained.[6]

§

This book is divided into three parts. In Part I, I establish a theoretical grounding for the book by exploring some of the large-scale "realities and myths" that govern our lives. In Part II, I share the real meaning behind the capacities of critical thinking that are the bedrock of development into the subjective state. And in Part III, I turn to three examples of subject-activation to explore three additional virtues needed to bring the subjective self to life: honesty, patience, and bravery. I conclude with a few reflections on the value of thinking.

What I do *not* offer here are step-by-step instructions on how to conduct critical thinking or how to be more honest, patient, and brave. These are necessary steps in the journey toward subjectivity, yet delivering them as *instructions* or *guidelines* would be self-contradictory and futile, since it would mean telling readers to follow rules, orders, and commands according to my own authority. This process, rather than encouraging subjectivity, would turn readers into unthinking, task-following objects. Instead, I wish to treat every potential reader as a subject or potential subject, so I have adopted a *facilitative* approach, one that does not tell people to do this or that but, rather, offers ideas, examples, stories, and frameworks into which the reader can enter creatively, as a thinking subject.

The most I can say by way of prescription is this: If you wish to reach the subjective state, or to reach it more often or more profoundly, you may have to let go of some deep-seated myths about yourself and the world. You may have to face transition, potentiality, and ambiguity (Part I). You may have to develop or further develop capacities associated with critical thinking, which is actually a radical kind of thinking. This is what I consider to be the fundamental building-block of the subjective state, so I spend a bit of time working through its details (Part II). Finally, you may have to practice honesty and, particularly, self-honesty, and you may have to find patience and bravery as you continue with your subjective practice (Part III).

If this is all too much for now and you wish to return to the first building block of developing subjectivity, I can recommend my book, *Critical Thinking and the Subject of Inquiry: Capacities, Resilience, and Power*.[7] There you will find a more detailed setting-out of ideas, propositions, and textual analyses that should help you begin your quest. In any case, I sincerely hope you find the resources you are searching for on your journey.

The Ailment

One day, when I was very sick, I recalled a funny story, one related by an ancient Daoist. When I dug it out of my bookshelves, I was surprised at how it resonated with my experience.

Here is the story. It is a Daoist parable, attributed to Lieh Tzu (of fourth-century BCE China) and known now as "The Ailment."[8]

> Lung Shu said to the physician Wen Chi, "Your art is subtle. I have an ailment; can you cure it?" The physician said, "I will do as you say, but first tell me about your symptoms." Lung Shu said, "I am not honored when the whole village praises me, nor am I ashamed when the whole country criticizes me. Gain does not make me happy, loss does not grieve me. I look upon life as like death, and see wealth as like poverty. I view people as like pigs, and see myself as like others. At home I am as though at an inn, and I look upon my native village as like a foreign country. With these afflictions, rewards cannot encourage me, punishments cannot threaten me. I cannot be changed by flourishing or decline, gain or loss; I cannot be moved by sorrow or happiness. Thus I cannot serve the government, associate with friends, run my household, or control my servants. What sickness is this? Is there a way to cure it?" The physician had Lung Shu stand with his back to the light while he looked into his chest. After a while he said, "Aha! I see your heart; it is empty! You are nearly a sage. Six of the apertures of your heart are open, one of them is closed. This may be why you think the wisdom of a sage is an ailment. It cannot be stopped by my shallow art."

Now, I am not claiming to be six-sevenths of the way toward being a Daoist sage, even though I felt a kinship with some of Lung Shu's "symptoms": his equanimity, his balance in the face of gain or loss, and his immunity to praise or blame.

The story was relevant to me because Lung Shu suffered from what he called "afflictions" and because he believed he had a grave "ailment." Perhaps the most basic point of the parable is that what is actually an "enlightened" experience bothers Lung Shu because he judges it to be unfortunate and negative because he has not claimed his feelings as part of *his subjective experience* of life.

Feeling indifferent about praise or criticism is not painful in itself. Indeed, it is closer to the absence of pain. Why is it that, on some level, we fear the absence of pain more than we fear pain, itself? I would encourage you to reflect on that for a moment. I'll try to explain this oddity in the next chapter.

For now, if we are able to think about the situation critically, we can see that it is the negative judgment attached to his experience along with Lung Shu's lack of subjective ownership of his experience that causes his suffering. Rather than embracing his feelings, Lung Shu decides he is *malfunctioning* in some way, that *there must be something wrong with him*. He no longer feels fear, but, paradoxically, his fearlessness is fearsome because it suggests to Lung Shu that he is broken, different, backwards, alone. He looks out at the world and sees people most unlike himself. Why is he the way he is? Mustn't there be "something wrong" with him?

Notes

1 The works of Brene Brown and Tara Brach, for instance, offer self-help projects that, at least on the surface, seem to counter this trend. In Chapter 2, I briefly note the need for subjectivity if one is to take up political critique or opposition against the "great machinery" of our collective lives. While it is not the focus of this book, it is one area that distinguishes this book from the works of Brown or Brach. That is, the kind of subjective state described here is, among other things, a decisive first step to avoiding what Herbert Marcuse called "repressive tolerance," where changes in the individual are readily absorbed by the "tolerant" socio-political system so as to avoid being damning critiques of or challenges to that system. See Herbert Marcuse, "Repressive Tolerance," in *A Critique of Pure Tolerance*, eds. Robert Paul Wolff, Barrington Moore Jr., and Herbert Marcuse (Boston: Beacon Press, 1969), 95–137.

2 Wallace Stevens, "How to Live. What to Do," in *The Collected Poems of Wallace Stevens* (New York: Vintage Books, 1990), 125–26.

3 Heinz Kohut, *The Restoration of the Self* (Chicago, IL: University of Chicago Press, 1977), 99.

4 On this note, readers may enjoy a couple of earlier works: Matthew H. Bowker, *Misinterest: Essays, Pensées, and Dreams* (Santa Barbara, CA:

Punctum Books, 2019); David P. Levine and Matthew H. Bowker, *The Destroyed World and the Guilty Self: A Psychoanalytic Study of Culture and Politics* (London: Phoenix Publishing, 2019).

5 All of this is not even to mention that the *alternative* to a world of subjects is a *de-subjectified world,* where persons are more like objects: acted *upon,* broken, traumatized, or at least helplessly vulnerable to others and/or "the Other."

6 See the *Introduction* to: Matthew H. Bowker and Amy Buzby, eds., *D.W. Winnicott and Political Theory: Recentering the Subject* (New York: Palgrave Macmillan, 2017); Matthew H. Bowker, *Ideologies of Experience: Trauma, Failure, Deprivation, and the Abandonment of the Self* (New York and London: Routledge, 2016); Matthew H. Bowker, "Activity, Speech, and Change: Progressive Politics and Regressive Fantasies," *Psychoanalysis, Culture & Society* 24, no. 2 (2019): 105–17; Matthew H. Bowker, "Analytic and Political Neutrality: Change, Privilege, and Responsibility," *Free Associations* 71 (2018): 1–17.

7 Matthew H. Bowker, *Critical Thinking and the Subject of Inquiry: Capacities, Resilience, and Power* (Redwood City, CA: Bluemount, 2025).

8 Thomas Cleary, *The Spirit of Tao* (Boston: Shambhala Publications, 1998), 73–74.

2 “Something Wrong”

What does it mean to feel that there is *something wrong* with us? In many cases, it simply means that we are different, traveling in a direction opposite to or orthogonal to (i.e., perpendicular to) the direction of the crowd.

One of the more radical steps taken by both “Eastern” and “Western” philosophies over the ages has been the willingness to consider the possibility that the crowd, the group, the society, or the other people in our world may *not* be heading in the right direction.

Among an ignorant crew that knows nothing of sailing, as one of Plato’s famous metaphors goes, the “true navigator” stands aside, calculating the wind and staring into the sky, appearing ludicrous to those who care only about gaining control of the vessel.

Among a band of fugitives, the saying goes, the person who stands still appears to be running away.

The point of these metaphors is that it is not necessarily a fault in the person if his, her, or their course diverges from society’s. The mass may be mistaken. The person may be enlightened.

Feeling that there is “something wrong” with us is often an internalization of (a “taking in” of) something that is wrong with the objects around us and our relationships with them. An insensitive friend or partner may leave one feeling that one is, instead, “hyper-sensitive,” and may send one off to the psychologist for help with this “symptom.” A chaotic and violent family life may make a child feel that he, she, or they are chaotic and violent inside. The objects whose properties we internalize may be our families, loved ones, work colleagues, or socio-cultural groups. Together, they compose the great machinery in which we live.

Internalizing the wrongness of part or all of the great machinery that surrounds us is a kind of coping mechanism, one often learned in childhood, when one lacked the wherewithal to perceive and point out what was “wrong” in a parent, teacher, boss, or social system. It is easier to find fault in oneself – because, theoretically, that fault can be corrected – than to find fault in the machinery. For one thing, we may idealize our parents, teachers, or leaders. Blaming ourselves allows us to keep those idealizations intact. The psychoanalyst Ronald

DOI: 10.4324/9781003626398-3

Fairbairn wrote famously that it feels better to be "a sinner in a world ruled by God than to live [as an innocent] in a world ruled by the Devil."[1] Only in the former situation is there hope. The world remains a good place; all is not lost.

For many years, I assumed that there was something terribly wrong with me. Not just with my body or outward life, but with my most inward being, my self, my soul. My mother used to have episodes of intense anger. One day, I was "nothing but a dumb f – ing jock." Most often, I was "rotten." I don't think I will ever be able to look at a rotting fruit or animal carcass without shivering. "Rotten" meant utterly ruined. What is rotten is foul and tainted to the very core. Part of my journey toward subjectivity (alluded to again in the context of psychoanalysis in Chapter 15) was facing up to these insulting characterizations, particularly the attribution of rottenness, to see where they came from, where they were, and where they truly belonged.

No well-meaning friend or psycho-therapist can sit you down and convince that you are not rotten. Well, they can try, but it does little good. To contend with a "wrongness" like this takes internal work and sustained subjective activity: thinking, remembering, questioning, working-through, facing fear and anxiety, again and again. For me to trust myself, to believe in myself, and to be myself meant that I had first to dislodge that rottenness. I had to replace my mother in the role of parent and re-teach myself about myself. If my mother had not died relatively young, I would have had to have had a frank conversation with her about rottenness. I've had the imaginary conversation with her, and it was fearsome enough.

So, placing the blame where it belongs is difficult and frightening, yet essential, if for no other reason than it allows us to know ourselves more fully, more realistically, such that we can be ourselves, become ourselves, even love ourselves. Knowing where to place "what is wrong" helps us to hold a more accurate view of our own past, present, and future, our reality and our potential. If we feel that there is something wrong with us, we are less likely and less able to undertake daring ventures, trust our instincts, and live creatively. Placing wrong where it belongs allows us to act, with respect to that wrongness, in a meaningful way: It tells us what, if anything, needs to be addressed and, possibly, corrected.[2]

You may not consider yourself a political person. In spite of my training in political science and in spite of having attended a handful of marches and protests, I do not consider myself anything like a political activist. Nevertheless, although this book is not expressly political in the sense that it does not offer *political* strategies for opposing or changing flaws in the socio-political machinery, it remains true that to be an effective political critic of the socio-political systems around us, one, first, has to be able to live as a subject. One has to be able to step back and *dis-internalize* individual suffering and symptoms to see them as sufferings and symptoms embedded in others, organizations, groups, ideologies, and societies. But this position comes with risks: One feels (and one may well be right) that one may lose the love or support of family, friends, or colleagues, not to mention social standing, a job, or career. One must have the resilience to weather immense psychological pressure, pressure that can make a person feel crazy, deviant, and more.[3]

§

In the words of Alexis de Tocqueville, the great scholar of American life in the nineteenth century, the public, in a modern democracy (such as the United States), comes to take on the quality of a king or a god. The reason why the public or the majority takes on this awe-inspiring aspect has to do with the internal logic of democracies, in which we believe that the people around us are, by and large, all created equal. If we did not believe this, then there would be no sense in democracy, since democracy means that the majority rules, that two heads are better than one, and that a majority of heads, if you will, is better than a minority. It is hard to defy the will of a great mass or majority of people if we also invest in them the greater part of sense or wisdom.[4]

For Tocqueville, the difficulty in thinking and acting contrary to the will of the public results from the fact that the public acts not on the body of the individual but on the mind or soul. In effect, the public whispers to the individual: "You can think how you like, but know that if you disagree with us, you will be alone, an alien, separated from the community you love."

In fact, even this statement misses the mark a bit, insofar as it makes it seem that we are fully aware of the social and psychological punishments that await us if we diverge from the group. In some cases, there are no real punishments at all: They are *mythical*. The threat of social punishment is embedded in us *unconsciously*, internalized as part of a lifelong education and socialization that begins in the family and is essentially a kind of training in how to be recognizable and likeable to others.

Thus, if it begins to dawn on us, one day, to think about a certain matter differently, we may experience it not as a clear alternative, a possibility we can choose or follow. Rather, we may find that our own intuitive, authentic thinking leads us quickly into a strange muddling of the mind, or a vague anxiety: enough to give us trouble composing our thoughts and returning us to whatever we had been occupied with before. Psychologically, we would speak about this experience as a block, or a site of resistance, where the individual is diverted from thoughts determined to be "dangerous" by an ever-watchful, protective part of our minds. Thus, as soon as the dangerous thought arises, it is kiboshed by confusion, or stress, or a vague sense of worry, irritation, or ennui.

What is really at issue, then, when we feel there is something "wrong" with us, is both a conscious fear of ostracism or punishment and an unconscious expression of the feeling that we have stepped out of an unmarked circle, wandered dangerously far from the group, lost sight of our family, community, or society, to which we must otherwise be devoted if we are to remain safe.

Understanding our conscious and unconscious resistances to divergent thinking helps us to understand why moving closer to our own subjectivity feels *scary*. It is frightening to feel at odds with our family, community, or society. Our imaginations of other people's disapproval carry us away and make us believe that we are broken, useless, maybe even a candidate for exile from the group.

Notes

1 W.R.D. Fairbairn, "The Repression and the Return of Bad Objects," in *Psychoanalytic Studies of the Personality* (London: Routledge & Kegan Paul, 1952), 67.
2 Here is where the development of realistic and healthy self-boundaries becomes an important step – a step associated with critical thinking, discussed in Part II – toward the critique of ideology and the potential for radical action.
3 For a fascinating study of these and other effects of opposing the "machinery," see C. Fred Alford, *Whistleblowers: Broken Lives and Organizational Power* (Ithaca, NY: Cornell University Press, 2001).
4 Alexis de Tocqueville, *Democracy in America*, trans. Harvey C. Mansfield and Delba Winthrop. (Chicago: University of Chicago Press, 2000).

3 The Fear of Freedom

Having said all of this, we can go one step deeper with Lung Shu. Recall that Lung Shu complains that "rewards cannot encourage me, punishments cannot threaten me. I cannot be changed by flourishing or decline, gain or loss; I cannot be moved by sorrow or happiness." Lung Shu knows that he has become removed from, even immune to, what we may think of as the pulleys and levers within the great machinery of social, economic, and cultural life. He finds that, instead, he is immovable.

Being immovable, Lung Shu stands apart. He is both grounded and free, and this experience frightens him terribly. He goes so far as to beg to be returned by the physician to a state where he can be *more* easily manipulated by reward and punishment. Imagine, again, how strange that is. Why should we long to be manipulated?

The answer is that if he cannot be pulled and pushed by good or bad, by pleasure or pain, by gain or loss, he is *out of control*. We might wish to think a bit more about that phrase and all it means to us. We rarely hear people speaking positively about someone or something that is "out of control." It has a distinctly negative connotation. The reason for that is because things that are out of control are unable to *function reliably* in the great machinery. From the perspective of the great machinery, they are dysfunctional elements, useless if not dangerous.

It is a fascinating puzzle that we, who so often long for freedom and independence, struggle when we find even a little of it. We fear what others will think about us and do to us if we break free and, in a phrase, "are left to our own devices." Being "left to our own devices" is another telling phrase that we typically hear with a distinctly negative slant, as in: "Left to his own devices, he'll likely fall apart," or "Left to her own devices, she'll never make the grade."

What these phrases are trying to tell us is that part of us fears freedom and *longs to be controlled.* Without having even explored or tested them, we judge that "our own devices" are not as trustworthy, not as good as the devices of society's great machinery. It is those devices, with all of their reliable pulleys and levers, that we can trust, not because they get us closer to the things we want but because, so long as we attach ourselves to the devices laid out for us

DOI: 10.4324/9781003626398-4

by our groups, we remain recognizable and loveable to them. We have a need rooted in a primal connection to our groups that expresses itself every time we feel afraid to set ourselves free from them. Let me say a word about this primal connection.

§

Humans have always lived in groups. In spite of myths and legends that teach otherwise – indeed, in spite of the Social Contract Theory that forms the bedrock of most modern, democratic constitutions – there never were free, solitary individuals roaming the Earth. Born into the family and the group, we are instantly and thoroughly dependent on others for our own survival.

As helpless infants and children, we could never make it on our own. What is more, to learn the ways, the customs, the rites, and the language of the group is to learn how to survive in the social world. We owe the group our lives.

We express this immeasurable debt when we align ourselves with our groups' ways of being and doing, when we share in the warmth of the embrace of the family, and when we feel a uniquely agonizing guilt for even thinking about stepping outside of the laws and principles that organize our communities.

If we fail to contribute to the group, or fail to hold a recognized and esteemed place within the group, we fear we will encounter the group's rejection. Since we have come to psychologically identify with the group – which means to see through its eyes and take on its judgment as our own – we become our own taskmasters, pushing ourselves to succeed on the group's terms, punishing ourselves should we ever fail to live up to the group's standards.

After doing this for most of our lives – in school, at work, in social encounters, and more – the recognition of the group is how we come to recognize ourselves. Our role in the group's great machinery is how we know who we are, where we stand, and what we are worth. We, ourselves, enforce this arrangement through self-imposed fear and guilt, even though it guarantees that genuine, spontaneous, subjective thoughts or actions will ring our alarm bells and quickly get shut down, since they could be indicative of impending dysfunction.

Lung Shu explains that, because he cannot be moved by the pulleys and levers that operate the group's great machinery, he "cannot serve the government, associate with friends, run [his] household, or control [his] servants." The consequence of dysfunctioning is the terribly fearsome sense that we can no longer contribute to our group(s) and are, therefore, in breach of our obligations, the performance of which keeps us alive and connects us with the world that sustains us.

4 The Great Machinery and the Myth of Human Mechanics

In the end, we must *dare to dysfunction*, but not because dysfunctioning is so wonderful in itself. On the contrary, it can be sad, scary, and painful. It can trigger tremendous losses. Nevertheless, in spite of its difficulty, we have to be willing to dysfunction if we are to be free. We have to achieve a stronger connection with ourselves than we have with the success or failure of the great social, cultural, political, and economic machinery. I hope that these messages become clearer as this chapter proceeds.

The underrated British anti-psychiatrist David Smail wrote, among other things, an extraordinary book called *Illusion and Reality: The Meaning of Anxiety*, which is not as complicated as it sounds.[1] The thrust of the work is an exposition of the idea that we have come to live in an objective world, to the detriment of the subjective.

The objective world is there, and it is needed: We have to have a shared, objective world to live and work together productively. But Smail turns the idea of objectivity into something more. He reminds us that the danger of living in an objective world is that we will come to mistake ourselves for objects, for things, for machines.

Machines function predictably and perform required tasks, assuming all is going normally. Thought of in this way, the objectively understood person functions and performs in order to secure a place in the great machinery that is well recognized and financially rewarding. This person, in his, her, or their objective role, is productive, healthy, physically attractive, sane, on good terms with family members and friends, and the like.

If we regard ourselves in this objective light, we are likely to find more than a few flaws: guilt-inducing aspects of ourselves that are failing to function perfectly. We may not be wealthy enough. We may not own a home. We may be having trouble completing tasks at work on time. We may be holding on to a few extra pounds or may not consider ourselves attractive. We may need psychological help to feel well. Our family relationships may not always be happy or harmonious. The list could go on.

Ultimately, when we define ourselves by our place in the great machinery of group life, we forget that our bodies are not machines, our minds are not

DOI: 10.4324/9781003626398-5

super-computers, and our selves are not robots. What I like to call the *myth of human mechanics* holds that, barring some identifiable and justifiable excuse, we ought to *function perfectly* in our jobs, our personal (physical and mental) health, and our social and domestic lives. The *myth of human mechanics* also holds that, if we ever cease to function perfectly, if we ever dysfunction, there must be something wrong with us as individuals and not with the machine. We must be the broken cogs. The machine is assumed to be flawless. There are several unfortunate consequences of this.

First, imagine what happens if we ever catch a whiff of difference or abnormality on our own part. Most of us hide it away. Abnormality suggests lack of fit. Lack of fit, like a misshapen cog, suggests dysfunctionality. Repeatedly shutting out our own natural thoughts, feelings, or impulses turns into a brutal and punishing aspect of our relationship with ourselves. We may call this relationship "self-discipline" or "vigilance" or whatever we like, but if, at its root, it is a blocking out of the abnormal, just because it is abnormal, then we are effectively excluding parts of ourselves from seeing the light of day. This kind of harsh self-repression can create severe depression, anxiety, and worse, as little pieces of ourselves and our nascent subjective experience are cast down into the abyss of the unconscious, where (we hope) no one will ever notice them.

Second, because the high standards we set for ourselves, according to the myth of human mechanics, are virtually impossible to meet, and because dysfunctioning is so scary and painful, we have little choice but to set up a phony, *false self* which impersonates the kind of mechanistic, super-computing, perfectly functioning object we believe we are supposed to be. This object (perhaps it is like an "artificial intelligence") – both in what it does and in what it does not do – satisfies others' needs and desires for us to be infallible, yet appropriately self-deprecating, stable, yet charming, and, although affable and lively when appropriate, impervious to the realities of human vulnerability, frailty, or change.

It is this *false self* we trot out most noticeably at job interviews, in early stages of relationships, or in other high-pressure moments of life when we want others to believe that we, too, are perfectly functioning objects that will never fail, and so will fit neatly well into whatever role in the machinery is on offer. Unfortunately, the false self is not just a mask we can so easily take on or off. It has staying power and can infiltrate even our most intimate relationships and activities. Although its origin is really an act of extreme compliance, it may become how we know and understand ourselves: our definitions, that is, of who we are.

Third, some part of us, however small, may catch us out. Even in subjectively underdeveloped persons, there is typically a small part of us that senses or knows intuitively that we are playing false, dressing ourselves up as perfect objects. On some level, maybe only in certain, special, reflective moments, we know that it is all an act. But once this knowledge rears its ugly head, we fall into an awful desperation, since we now must recognize that we are lying to ourselves and others. We do not stop and think critically enough about the situation to realize that everyone is playing the same game. Instead, we suffer "imposter syndrome" and a dread of being found out by people better than us. We are in a truly unfortunate situation, caught between playing an impossible role and feeling fear and guilt for being unable to play it perfectly.

§

It is a tragedy that, in our distress, we find it hard to summon a critical challenge to the myth of human mechanics, to assert our subjective freedom from the operations of the great machinery. It is perhaps even more tragic that, should we turn to a "helping professional" with our problems, we find very often that the helping professional is *part* of the great machinery, unable to see beyond the myth. All too often, when we seek "professional help" (and that includes a lot of "self-help"), we find encouragements to strengthen or refine our false selves, to become a more brilliant cog, rather than to set the *myth* aside, let the machinery break down, and get to know our real subjective selves.

Just think of the armies of professionals ready to assist you in fitting into the great machinery: psychiatrists, psychologists, doctors, life coaches, influencers, social workers, teachers, religious advisers, cosmetic surgeons, financial planners, beauticians, accountants . . . The list could go on and on. In most cases, such professionals aim to fix what seems to be dysfunctioning in you and to fit you back into society, not to stand alongside you and assert your right to be your own imperfect self. "In other words," Smail writes, "when you fail [to be a perfect object] you will find almost no one ready to take your failure seriously, and no conceptual structure, no language, in which to consider it – you will just be exhorted to try even harder to succeed."[2]

Let's return once again to the position of Lung Shu. Should he, instead of having met with the physician Wen Chi, have met with a contemporary psychiatrist or doctor of some sort, the ending of the parable would have been very different. Rather than seeing Lug Shu's predicament as one of near-wisdom, of near-freedom from social and cultural dependence, and of a grounded *being*, Lung Shu would likely have ended up in a course of CBT (cognitive behavioral therapy) with a diagnosis of "Major Depression."

§

Because we have set up a false self, and because others have so as well, we inhabit a false self *system* that is best described as *mythical*. Not grounded in authentic experience or critical thought about that experience, the mythical world is a game of pretend that has gotten out of hand and has become distinctively cruel. This is because, in order to pass muster in the world of objectified selves, it is not enough to turn ourselves in to perfectly functioning objects: We must continually pursue and obtain recognition by others as just such objects.

> We come to depend, as a matter of survival,
>
> on the presence of others who will accord us validity, identity and reality. You cannot be anything if you are not recognized as something; in this way your being becomes dependent on the regard of somebody else. You may be confirmed, or you may be disconfirmed, and if the latter is the case often enough and pervasively enough, you simply cease to exist as a person.[3]

Because of the myth of human mechanics, we end up an object in a world of objects, trying desperately to convince other objects we imagine to be perfect that we, too, are perfect. It is worth a moment to pause and consider how insane this quest is. We become deeply vulnerable to failure and guilt as we depend, for our lives and identities, on the opinions of objectifying others.

Although we think the way to escape is to succeed, to "win" the game or "beat the machine," as it were, that is an inherently flawed proposition. We can never have or do enough to break free of the sense that we ought to be perfect but are not. We cannot break free until we give up the never-ending chase for perfect functionality and treat ourselves as subjects. It is only as subjects that we find hope for resilience, groundedness, and freedom from the mythical world. It is to that possibility I now turn.

Notes

1 David Smail, *Illusion and Reality: The Meaning of Anxiety* (London: J.M. Dent & Sons, 1984).
2 Smail, *Illusion and Reality*, 15.
3 Smail, *Illusion and Reality*, 18.

5 Realities

Over the past several years, if I were to regard myself an object, I could only conclude that I was dysfunctioning. My physical and mental health were suffering; my work life was threatened; my sources of both productivity and income were highly vulnerable. As an object, I was breaking or broken.

Looking at myself as a subject, however, things were less bleak. I could still think, dream, and create. (I could create lectures for classes and books and papers to be published.) I could still be with my family and give and receive love. I could still be myself. I could be *with* myself and remain in a state of subjective self-contact.

This is where I believe a lot of popular self-help goes wrong, particularly if it is infused with "Western" understandings of "Eastern" traditions. There are several traditions of thought, largely coming from what we refer to as "the East" (typically meaning Asia), in which the goal seems to be to get rid of the self. Conflated with the ego, which is, itself, a misunderstood construct, the self appears to many to be what stands in the way of inner peace. Get rid of the self, get rid of the ego, the teachings promise, and you will become one with the world, with nature, or with the universe.

I think the situation is vastly more subtle. After all, we are still human *beings*. To get rid of our unique *being*, in order to think of ourselves as mere things floating through space, does a disservice to our specialness and subjectivity, our unique opportunity to *be* human and to *be* who we are.

At the same time, such teachings misunderstand the nature of objective reality. In objective reality, what stands out as most important is that there is a world that is *not me*. There is a reality, full of other, separate objects, with which I will never be fully one.

One way to read the teachings of, say, ancient Daoism, is to see them as paradoxes: paradoxes that must remain paradoxes in order to impart their full wisdom. The wisdom of one Daoist paradox is that we can inhabit a space where we both *are* and *are not*, where we are our complete selves, and yet are also just a bit of scenery. There is a way to exist as both subjects and objects.

DOI: 10.4324/9781003626398-6

The "Reality Principle"

As I have tried to show in the foregoing chapters, no matter how great our efforts to fortify our false selves, we never escape the myth of human mechanics or the great machinery of the world by doing so. We can spend a lifetime trying to build up a false self that is invulnerable in the objective world, so rich that it could never be thought poor, so smart that it could never be thought dumb. This, I have argued, is an endless chase, for it is the nature of the myth and the machinery that we always rediscover our conditionality: the fact that, in the objective world, we live and die by the regard of others.

What is more, if we were not fortunate enough to have been the recipient of unconditional love as children or young adults (and many of us were not), we now find it agonizing that love is the currency of approval or disapproval, confirmation or disconfirmation. Conditional love can be given or taken away. When taken away, it is as if we do not exist. We die. The threat of the loss of love, which so many of us fear, only really applies in the world of objects.

Some of us have, I think, put love to a great misuse, making it conditional, loving people as objects rather than as subjects. Love has come to signify a certain kind of approval, a confirmation of an object that meets certain objective criteria. Because people cover us up with objective labels that describe what we *are* – I love Jane because Jane *is* good, or smart, or strong – we have to continually earn the love of others by becoming and remaining the kinds of objects they find us and want us to be.

What we have so far referred to as the objective world is part of what psychoanalysts call "The Reality Principle."[1] The Reality Principle is, like the objective world, necessary but not sufficient to have a meaningful life.

Let's think developmentally: Infants typically begin without any understanding of how reality works. This is part of the magic of being an infant: It is close to a completely subjective experience of reality because the whole world seems to revolve around the infant's feelings, fantasies, and impulses. Most infants, if they are cared for adequately, begin by believing that they are all-powerful masters of the universe, for when they are hungry, food appears, and when they are upset, they are hugged and comforted.

Gradually, as parents' abilities to adapt to their children's increasingly complex needs wane, children discover that they are not omnipotent but occupy only a limited place in reality, a reality that includes others, where others have needs and duties and feelings and projects that are equal in importance to, if not at times superior in importance to, those of the children. Infants who began as subjective gods at the center of their own universes come to discover, one day, that to be hugged requires another, separate person to come and hug them.

At this point, children have to confront and, hopefully, accept the Reality Principle, in order to continue developing. The Reality Principle teaches us that there are things in the world that are not under our control, that are not subject to our wish and whim, that there are others in the world of equal importance to us, that our actions have consequences, that we are not gods. Although it comes across as a kind of insult to the omnipotence of the infant, I cannot emphasize enough how important it is for a child to be able to accept the Reality Principle.

At the same time, if the Reality Principle is introduced too soon, or to harshly, it can crush the soul of a child, whose subsequent life will show signs of almost nothing but adaptation to external stimuli, which is to say, almost nothing but *objective* being and doing. Where will the child have gone? No one knows. But clearly, the "real" world of others will have, sadly, become all-important and the "imaginary" world of the infant will have been eclipsed, along with the nascent becoming of a whole, healthy, subjective person.

What it takes to navigate the Reality Principle is an appreciation for paradox, an ability to hold onto infantile magic while, at the same time, recognizing the real, objective difference of others and of the world. The British psychoanalyst, Donald Winnicott, argued that paradox could be appreciated best in what he called *transitional space* or, sometimes, *potential space*. Transitional space is a somewhat complex concept, but, at its root, it refers to a possibility of experiencing life both subjectively and objectively, as connected to both the inner world and the outer world, and as straddling the domains of what is *me* and what is *not me*. It is here, Winnicott thought, that creativity, play, symbolism, and cultural life occur.[2]

Transitional and Potential Reality

There is a poem I loved from my youth that I also used to read to my daughter when she was little. Indeed, it comes from the volume, *When We Were Very Young*, by A.A. Milne, the creator of the *Winnie the Pooh* tales. The poem is called "Halfway Down" and goes like this:

> Halfway down the stairs
> Is a stair
> Where I sit.
> There isn't any
> Other stair
> Quite like
> It.
> I'm not at the bottom,
> I'm not at the top;
> So this is the stair
> Where
> I always
> Stop.
> Halfway up the stairs

Isn't up
And isn't down.
It isn't in the nursery,
It isn't in the town.
And all sorts of funny thoughts
Run round my head:
"It isn't really
Anywhere!
It's somewhere else
Instead!"[3]

Milne is describing something very special indeed. It is a treasured place, that certain stair that is both and neither upstairs nor downstairs, both and neither in the subjective world of fantasy the child might associate with the nursery nor in the objective world of grown-ups and serious things the child might associate with being in the town. That stair is the child's transitional and potential space. And having or finding a transitional and potential space is critical for the child to be able to *build bridges* between his, her, or their inner, subjective world and the objective, "real" world outside.

The child who sits on the certain stair is, by being in-between, able to experience both reality and imagination, both the familiar and the unknown, both everywhere and nowhere, both the world and the self. Because the certain stair is, in one sense, a *no-place*, it opens up for the child the possibility of being *any place*, of being both places or even all places all at once.

When I reflected on my own reactions and feelings about life over the past several years, I recognized that things had been very difficult, but I also sensed that I was, in some ways, returning more and more frequently to that certain stair. On that certain stair, I was in between peace and crisis, fulfillment and need, happiness and sadness, openness and closure.

All of this is not to say that I was stuck in the middle. The experience was very nearly the opposite. I found myself somewhere where anything seemed possible, even though possibilities were being scratched off, cut off, day by day, given what was happening to me. I felt sad and happy at the same time, and, most importantly, my feelings felt real and, I dare say, *dear* to me, even if they were partly painful. Wherever I was between good and bad, fortune and misfortune, I felt a powerful sense of aliveness that let me know that my feelings reflected a subjective standing.

Enlightened or Depressed?

A couple of years ago, in the midst of one of my illnesses, and having just returned to work from a short stay in the mental hospital, I walked into a seminar I was teaching on autoethnographic writing. I sat down. I looked out at the students and we all remained silent for a few minutes, as usual.

Finally, I asked, "How are you?"

The students responded with varying degrees of "Well," until one asked me, boldly: "Are you enlightened or are you depressed?"

I was a little surprised. I had to pause and reflect on the question.

She continued, "because you have such a calming presence and I like coming to this class because it really relaxes me. You seem very . . . at peace. But, then again, depression can express itself this way. You know? Like, it can look like that."

Her explanation made sense and, in its attention to my subjectivity and my emotional state, it was intimate. So we all sat and thought for a little while. Because of the intimacy of the question, and because of the intimacy I try to create in my seminars, the silence did not feel threatening.

Eventually, I said, "Well, thank you for asking. I understand what you mean. But I'm not sure. Maybe it's *both.*"

This elicited a lot of laughter from the group, and from me, in part because of the *apparently* obvious contradiction between being "at peace" and being "depressed," and in part because I had just raised the possibility that I, myself, was "enlightened."

In fact, the correct answer *was* "both." I *was* depressed. I had just been released from the hospital for depression. And I was taking lots of medications to address my depression, some of which, I suspect, made me even more depressed, while others made me feel crazy in other ways. I was depressed, even though I was fortunate enough to teach bright, young people.

At the same time, maybe being "depressed" – whatever that means – was part of being "enlightened" – whatever that means. I certainly don't think that's out of the question. Even an enlightened take on objective reality can be depressing, as we witness the great sufferings of others. Enlightened people can also have subjective experiences in which they are, for whatever reason, depressed.

What stood out to me about this interaction is that the students were able to perceive both my "depression" and my "enlightenment." My subjective presence in the group, in which I felt connected to my true being, brought with it a warmth, stillness, and calm for students, where the normal worries of objective approval or disapproval, liking or disliking, passing or failing, did not arise. I had a way of being with students that made our interactions feel honest and even special. By being a subject in their presence, I facilitated their development as subjects and they facilitated mine.

It helped that, when I entered a classroom, even if I felt ill, I resonated with a lofty purpose: the purpose of higher education. This purpose was and remains sacred to me. It has to do with facilitating students' subjectivities so that they can explore, learn, and grow as persons. Facilitation – and we'll talk more about facilitation in the coming chapters – also means letting go of the desire to put on a learned, false front or to just bestow my knowledge on students, both of which are usually narcissistic desires that reflect a teacher's need to create, then witness, little versions of their own knowledgeable selves in students.

The student had discovered and revealed, although without knowing it, that the classroom was a transitional or potential space. It was a place where I was myself while also being what students needed me to be. It was a place where we had objective tasks to complete, readings to discuss, and the like, but it was also a space for subjective interactions between persons. In this space, our discussions were open, intimate, and comfortable. There was ample room for deep critical thinking to take place. Because of the way that the transitional space made room for subjectivities to come to life, the students' work seemed to happen spontaneously, genuinely, even effortlessly. The *Dao De Jing* says that when the teacher's work is done, "the people say, 'Amazing: we did it, all by ourselves!'"[4] That sounds about right.

Notes

1 Sigmund Freud, *Beyond the Pleasure Principle*, trans. James Strachey (New York: W.W. Norton & Company, 1961).
2 D.W. Winnicott, "Transitional Objects and Transitional Phenomena," in *Playing and Reality* (London: Tavistock Publications, 1971), 1–25.
3 A.A. Milne, *When We Were Very Young* (New York: Dutton, 1924).
4 Stephen Mitchell, trans., *Tao Te Ching* (New York: Harper & Row, 1988, Chapter 17).

6 Subjects and Objects

If teaching is about facilitating the development of students' subjectivities, we must know what it means to be a subject, to inhabit a subjective state. What follows was, and is, my clearest understanding of what it means to be a subject and, conversely, what it means not to be a subject.

First and foremost, a subject *is*. A subject is a *being* and is capable of *being* without a lot of props or supports from the world of others and of external stimuli. This is the subject's relative (not absolute) autonomy.

A lot has been written lately about people's experiences of solitude or being alone. I have contributed a bit to this literature in trying to convey that a rich experience of being alone is really a subjective capacity, that many people fail to *be* when they are alone, and that, of course, many people run from the experience of solitude precisely because it threatens something about their sense of themselves.

It is important to note that a subject is a person who thinks and acts for himself, herself, or themselves, not in the sense of being egotistical or selfish, but in that what a subject thinks and does (at least much of the time) emanates from impulses, decisions, and cognitive and emotional processes that are *internal* to the person.

Put another way, a subject's thoughts, words, and deeds are not mere reactions to stimuli, nor are they robotic repetitions of something memorized. Instead, they are *creative*, in that they are "created" internally by him, her, or them: They emanate from the subject's core self or true being.[1]

Therefore, I think we can say that a basic definition of a subject is a relatively *autonomous and capacious person* for whom possibilities of thinking and doing are not unduly limited. A subject is a person who *is*, and who has the capacity to *do*. Indeed, a subject is a person for whom *what is done* arises naturally out of who he, she, or they *are*. A subject is a creature whose *doings* arise out of his, her, or their *being*.[2]

§

The development of subjects, in this sense, is or ought to be the fundamental goal of modern civilization. Certainly, it is a central goal of enlightened

DOI: 10.4324/9781003626398-7

parenting and teaching. And any course or training in which advanced thinking is a learning outcome must devote at least some of its time to helping individuals to enhance or enrich their subjecthood, introducing learners to the challenges associated with subjecthood, and reminding individuals and groups of the value of the subjective state.

The most common understanding of the term "subjective" is "opinion-based." And this is for a good reason. It is impossible to separate the critical capacities of a subject from his, her, or their ability to root thoughts, beliefs, and judgments in the *inner world*, in internal dynamics, even in fantasy. These subjective mental activities are, in an important sense, *disconnected* from "objective" reality, and they must be so. It is for this reason that objectively oriented people, some scientists, and those who represent the myth of human mechanics and the great machinery alluded to above are suspicious of "subjective" viewpoints.

But in truth, while there are times when we prefer an objective viewpoint to a subjective viewpoint, as in a debate about the scientific method, we could not exist meaningfully without subjective activities. We would not want to eliminate subjective viewpoints from our world any more than we would want to eliminate the imagination of new possibilities, dreaming dreams, conceptualizing things not yet in existence, or wishing for something to happen in the future.

In many branches of psychoanalytic theory, the terms "subject" and "object" map fairly closely onto the terms, "self" and "other." If one has reached a stage of maturity in which one's self has developed into an autonomous agent, capable of thinking and acting in ways that accord with authentic desires, impulses, and opinions, then one can be considered a "subject" who lives amidst and has relations with "objects" (other people).

In this language, "objects" are separate persons who are also "subjects" in their own right – or, at least, one is capable of treating them as such. For these others, one is a psychoanalytic "object" and yet, one hopes, one will be treated as a "subject," as an independent person who deserves respect and regard as an autonomous being in the world.

§

Needless to say, the project of developing subjecthood can go awry. *Persons can fail to become subjects*: Human beings can remain forever in a state of underdeveloped subjecthood, where they do not or cannot think or act for themselves, but, rather, depend upon others, on groups, on dogmas, on authority figures, or on other internal forces (which typically represent powerful others) to tell them what to think, how to live, and what to do.

What I have just mentioned is the main reason this book cannot be a step-by-step guide to becoming a subject: because such guides cast readers in unthinking roles, asking them to follow instructions and to rely on authority, rather than facilitating their capacity to think for themselves.

When someone fails to be a subject, it impacts not only that person but also others with whom that person relates. These others will *not* be treated as separate subjects or autonomous agents, but as something less, as characters in the underdeveloped subject's internal dramas, or as "mere objects" (in the sense of "inanimate objects") with no real agency of their own, objects that can be pushed and pulled along a prescribed path, to fit into the underdeveloped subject's world.

There is a kind of tragedy, perhaps the greatest tragedy, in a human being's incapacity to be a subject: when a human being fails, for one reason or another – and sometimes due to circumstances or disadvantages that are beyond the person's control – to achieve subjectivity. When the thoughts and actions of individuals or groups are determined by factors that are not consonant with autonomous, capacious selves, then, we might say, those individuals or groups are more *objects* than *subjects*.

Just using the term *subject*, therefore, does not presume that all persons are subjects, that subjecthood is easy to attain, nor even that subjecthood is perfectly or absolutely attainable. Nevertheless, it is immensely helpful to see the world through this lens: subjects and objects.

You are welcomed, even encouraged, to wonder whether, in fact, subjects and objects can be so easily distinguished or categorized. Some facets of human experience seem to suggest the opposite: that persons and groups shift or slide, if you will, back and forth between subject and object, often residing in the gray areas in between.

I would only reply that these *ideal* or *archetypal* distinctions do not in any way discount the reality of the blurriness between subject and object, and that the categories are *conceptually helpful*, even if they are hard to define or even mixed up in our real-life experiences. Indeed, becoming aware of the fine and often blurry lines between subject and object, between the modes of being that define both and the ease with which one may swing from one to the other, and between the factors and forces that facilitate subjecthood versus those that pull us toward objecthood are important parts of the journey.

As I will address in the next part of the book, we have to be able to develop certain basic capacities in order to come alive as subjects. I have grouped a few of the central capacities here under the heading: *critical thinking*. Put simply, the capacity for critical thinking works to the extent that we can:

- filter information,
- delineate and defend psychic boundaries, i.e. set limits as to what "gets in" and what "gets pushed out,"
- reflect on and sometimes resist familial, political, social, and other psychological pressures, and
- reflexively contemplate how one is thinking.

In order to pursue even greater subjective capacities, such as the capacity for genuine honesty, patience, and bravery, it is necessary to begin with the following building blocks. I hope you will find that analyzing them here helps you to develop your own subjective strength.

Notes

1 To take a step further, they are not reified or ossified in any particular state, time, or place as a fixed entity, even as the fixed entity called the "true self." On this point, Jeffrey Rubin's chapter "Does the True Self Really Exist?" is enlightening. (Jeffrey Rubin, *A Psychoanalysis for Our Time: Exploring the Blindness of the Seeing I* (New York: NYU Press, 1998), 99–113.)

2 See on this point: Donald W. Winnicott, *Home Is Where We Start From: Essays by a Psychoanalyst*, eds. Clare Winnicott, Ray Shepherd, and Madeleine Davis (New York: W.W. Norton & Company, 1986), 35–54.

Part II

Critical Thinking Is Radical Thinking

7 What Is Critical Thinking?

I recently came across a popular self-help book that advertised itself to consumers by promising that, if they followed along a prescribed path and completed all the exercises in the book, they would end up being more creative. "What a thoroughly *uncreative* way to try to become creative!," I thought. I sincerely doubt that anyone can develop deep and meaningful creativity in this way. They may develop tricks, or even skills, that can be applied creatively to various situations, but the followers of this program are not likely to find the kind of genuine, spontaneous, authentic, creative *doing* that arises naturally out of subjective *being*.[1]

So, once again, I don't have exercises for you. If you want exercises for developing your critical thinking abilities, you will find that they are readily available on the internet, in courses and training programs, or elsewhere. You will be told that practicing critical thinking involves things like:

- analyzing data,
- posing questions,
- seeking alternatives,
- evaluating or judging claims,
- reflecting on assumptions,
- and generating "out of the box" ideas.

You will find, in other words, a list of cognitive skills or processes that you can apply to a variety of situations. If that is what you want, it is all well and good.

But how helpful is a list like this for someone seeking to come into himself, herself, or themselves as a mature, developed subject? Not very. You can exercise all of the skills and processes you want and still find it impossible to adopt a subjective stance as a way of being in the world.

I have titled this book, *The Power of Being a Subject: Transcending Human Mechanics with Critical Thinking, Honesty, Patience, and Bravery*, for what I hope will be obvious reasons. Of these terms, the one we need to address right now is "critical thinking."

DOI: 10.4324/9781003626398-9

In spite of the watering down of critical thinking that has taken place since the concept took hold in higher education several decades ago, critical thinking is actually quite radical.[2] What I mean by "radical" is two things: First, I mean "radical" in the usual sense of being transformative, far-reaching, and revolutionary. Critical thinking has the power to upset and overturn what is uncritically thought, which informs a lot of what we do. Second, the word radical means "root," as the Latin root for the word "radical" is *radix*. Something that is radical gets to the root, the core, the foundation. Radical thoughts create *profound* perspectives. A radical thought examines a deep foundation thoroughly and maybe upsets what rests upon it.

The kind of thinking I describe in this section is radical: It is critical thinking that takes you to the roots of your own ideas, to address them at their deepest level, and maybe even to challenge the fundamental assumptions or paradigms supporting them. This kind of thinking, then, is the foundation for the possibility of a radical transformation into a subject state that this book recommends.

§

Asking the question, "What is critical thinking?", leads us into a minor paradox because, if we are too rigid in our approach to answering it, we will no longer be doing the right kind of work. That is, the more we strive to "pin down" or "settle on" a firm definition, the more we are tempted to stop investigating it: in order words, to be done with *thinking*.

Of course, no one would say that, in order to do the work of critical thinking, we have to avoid discovering answers. But we ought to be aware of the temptations to find *easy* answers, to find answers *prematurely*, or to consider our answers to be *final*. Such temptations typically express discomfort with ambiguity, a discomfort with which those who seek to enhance their capacities to think critically will have to contend.

For these reasons, I have found it helpful, over decades of study, teaching, and writing, to begin by imagining critical thinking *not* as a "thing," but as *a set of internal processes that compose a subjective capacity*.

The capacity that comprises the processes involved with critical thinking is not static, like a "skill" one learns and never forgets, but is, rather, fluid, dynamic, and ongoing. In this way, instead of asking what critical thinking *is*, we ought to ask what critical thinking *does*.

If we can do so, we will imagine the work of critical thinking in less absolute terms and more as the task of engaging subjective capacities that can be relatively active or relatively dormant, that can be bolstered or impaired, enhanced or forestalled. These subjective capacities need to be facilitated, engaged with, and reflected upon throughout life.

§

If critical thinking *does*, rather than *is*, what does it *do*? What are these "internal processes" by which critical thinking has just been defined?

By "internal," I mean anything that happens inside the mind or psyche of an individual, anything that happens within that person's psychic boundaries. So, these processes include questioning, concentrating, judging, and even blocking out what is distracting and/or unwanted.

To say that critical thinking describes a set of *internal processes* means that it involves the activation of complex capacities inside of us, capacities that support our existence as *the subject* – the creator or the author – of our own lives.

To activate and make use of these capacities without undue difficulty or interference is absolutely necessary if one wishes to be a subject. In order to be a subject, to put it simply and bluntly, one must possess the capacity *to think for oneself.* In turn, thinking for oneself entails thinking about, questioning, wondering about, and judging the extent to which the self can be determined by itself and by its own internal work of thinking.

If that last sentence seems a bit mysterious, perhaps an explanation is warranted. Not all parts of the self can be determined by the self alone, nor by thinking alone. One does not choose one's genetic makeup, one's birth parents, one's initial living environment, one's native language, race, ethnicity, place of origin, or sex at birth. One may not have freedom or choice over the many factors that may influence one's development in life. These factors include the presence or absence of certain other people, the social structures, political institutions, and powerful groups with which one is involved, and even the natural environment of which one forms a part.

At the same time, critical thinking is not, as some would have us imagine, mainly a question of "how to keep one's feet dry in a flood." The question of how to keep one's feet dry involves *instrumental* thinking (i.e., how to get from A to B, where B is a predetermined and unquestioned goal), which is not to say that it is not a very important question. It involves practical reasoning and planning, and can be of great service or utility.

Critical thinking, in the sense of the term pursued throughout this book, is not really oriented toward this kind of *practical* work. Rather, critical thinking prompts us to ask ourselves the following kinds of questions, which could be rather easily adapted and applied to a variety of situations other than a flood:

- How shall we situate ourselves in relation to the flood and its aftermath?
- Do we conceive of ourselves as victims or as agents with respect to it?
- How do we regard the flood? What baggage are we loading it with?
- How and to what extent do our pre-existing thought patterns and emotions, our pasts and our vulnerabilities, determine our courses of action or reaction?
- How much should we allow the flood to affect us, our states of mind, our internal and external lives?
- And, perhaps most importantly, will we permit the flood to diminish our subjecthood, such that we become, perhaps even if only for a time, mere *objects*, reacting and responding to overwhelming stimuli?

This example of the flood I have invoked mainly to suggest that critical thinking is both more and less than a “skill” or “tool” to help us navigate the practical difficulties associated with accidents, troubles, or other forces and factors that impact our lives. Critical thinking involves thinking about *how* to think about these contingencies, and, with them, how to think about human experience.

Notes

1 Indeed, I would argue that creative thinking is rooted in critical thinking, but that is unfortunately beyond the scope of this chapter.
2 If you are interested in the history of the idea of critical thinking, beyond my book, *Critical Thinking and the Subject of Inquiry* referenced above, I can also recommend a shorter article: Matthew H. Bowker and K. Patrick Fazioli, “Rethinking Critical Thinking: A Relational and Practical Approach,” *Pedagogy and the Human Sciences* 6, no. 1 (2016): 1–26.

8 Paradigms

Critical thinking means making contact with what is "inside" our minds, but it also means getting ourselves "outside" of what may be called "givens": pre-formed and/or established perspectives, sets of beliefs, ideologies, and *paradigms*, which are broad means of seeing and comprehending the world.

A paradigm is a kind of mental foundation and framework upon which we build our more detailed understandings of the world. Like a house, the foundation and framework are there to support and to provide structure for everything else. After we have built the foundation and framework, we can talk about hanging the walls and putting up the roof, running the plumbing and electricity and even establishing the décor. So the foundation and framework makes it possible to build a house, but it also limits us because we cannot build a house that does not fit the specifications of our foundation or framework. Similarly, a paradigm helps us to build a basic vision or understanding of life: how things work, why things happen, what we should do, and more.

There are no easy answers to the questions we will raise or to the confusion we will feel when we critically examine our own paradigms. There may be answers for us, but those answers will *not* be absolute, certain, or automatic. Why? Because easy answers come from *within* paradigms, whereas we are trying to examine the paradigms themselves, to better analyze, comprehend, and compare them.

§

In life, we need paradigms. We regularly operate within them and, frankly, *we can't live without them*, although we rarely consciously choose them. The trick is to recognize that we live and operate inside paradigms and to be able to see their origins, limitations, and consequences. The goal is to recognize the assumptions, beliefs, and prejudices that are *built into* our paradigms, often without our being aware.

To recognize *that* we (collectively although not always consciously) choose and *how* we (collectively although not always consciously) choose paradigms within which to think, act, and relate requires that we see the underlying criteria

DOI: 10.4324/9781003626398-10

and values by which the paradigms have been chosen and, simultaneously, the underlying criteria and values propounded by our paradigms.

Let us say a person believes strongly in the value of science. He or she is impressed with scientific accomplishments and respects scientific authority. This person might ask himself, herself, or themselves: "Why believe in science?" And the answer may be: "Well, science *works*." And it's true: Science solves problems, creates technological progress, and the like.

However, now this person must ask:

- Why do I believe in and care about "what works"?
- Why do I believe in and care about "technological progress"?
- Is it because "what works" . . . *works* for me and because without "progress" . . . there would be *no progress* for me?
- What is the real value of "what works"? That is, as scholars famously ask utilitarians, what is the utility of utility?

Paradigms often lead us in circles.

Consider this another way: "Paradigm problems" cannot be solved in the same way mathematics problems can be solved. For paradigm problems, there is no "right" answer. In mathematics, one assumes a rational, mathematical paradigm and operates within. In critical thinking, the paradigm, itself, is not given but is *held in question.*

As we consider it, we may remark ourselves dipping in and out of other familiar paradigms, latching on to our second-favorite paradigm, or giving up hope altogether because we recognize that, in some sense, unless we can settle on a paradigm, we can never arrive at a certain conclusion. (Of course, then we must ask: Why is it so important to arrive at a "certain conclusion"?)

This last option – giving up hope – would, of course, be unfortunate, since the problems paradigms raise do not need to be *solved,* only observed, considered, and held in question in our minds. This can be quite difficult for those who need, for one reason or another, to approach life as a set of problems to be solved, obstacles to be overcome, or questions requiring answers. Such an orientation to life – seeing the world as if it were a math problem to be solved with finality – is, of course, reflective of an extremely rationalistic and scientific paradigm, meaning that those who adopt this paradigm are implicitly endorsing both the values and the limitations of that way of being, acting, and relating in the world.

§

I'd like to present a few examples of paradigm-conflict to show just how hard it is for paradigms to speak with other or outside paradigms. What I discovered in doing this work, in thinking like this about paradigms, is that many of us have multiple paradigms available to us at any given time. We can have internal arguments about things in our lives that depend heavily on which paradigm we select to hold the ideas together. In fact, I would venture to say that many of the hardest problems or puzzles we face as we age are problems of paradigm-clash, where we simply can't or don't know how to choose between paradigms.

To call these perspectives "paradigms" is to stretch the meaning of the term a little. These are small examples that we can talk about, but paradigms are, really, quite "large," encompassing whole cultures and societies. And again: Paradigms are shared. Their shared quality is exactly what gives paradigms their strength.

The following examples are, of course, highly simplified. I still believe, however, that we can see in them, instead of two or more persons, two or more parts of our selves, struggling to have a coherent argument with ourselves over an important issue. I would encourage you to reflect on these as you read them and see if any of them remind you of an internal dialogue or polylogue you have going on internally.

1. Jake, a precocious child, wants to eat a large chocolate cake instead of his dinner. His mother, Donna, tells him he may not. Jake says, "I don't care what is healthy. It is more important in life to eat what tastes good." Donna says, "No, it is more important to eat healthfully." Jake replies, "No, health is important to you but taste is important to me!" Donna tries to settle it: "I am your mother. I know best. You will see when you get older." But Jake explains, "When I get older, I will also think I know best, and I will tell my kids to eat healthfully, but I will be wrong then because I am right now. If you could grow younger, you would see."
2. Henry sits down with his parole officer, Susan. Susan asks Henry, "Have you come to understand that your crime was morally wrong?" Henry responds, "No, stealing that money was right because I needed it to survive. What is 'wrong' is that I faced a situation in which, owing to no fault of my own, I needed to steal just to live." Susan argues, "There is no excuse for committing crimes." Henry replies, "There are many valid excuses for committing crimes: self-defense, civil disobedience, civic protest. When the law is unjust, it is just to break the law." Susan retorts, "But the law is not unjust." Henry says, "I guess it depends on how you define 'just'."
3. Mike has an alcohol-abuse problem. His friend, Steve comes over to his apartment to conduct an intervention. Steve pleads with Mike, "You must stop drinking. You are ruining your life. You are miserable. You look terrible. You are risking your health, your relationships, your future, everything." Mike answers, "No, I am happy. Even though it might not seem so to you, I am happier than I have ever been. Drinking makes me really happy." Steve says, "Drinking is not real happiness." Mike asks, "What makes you think that you know any better than I do what real happiness is?" Steve answers, "Because I have a sober perspective."
4. Ann points to a basketball. She says to her young nephew Tom, "This is a basketball. It is orange." Tom says, "No, it is brown." Ann tries to persuade

Tom that the color of a basketball is more similar to the other things we call "orange" than to the things we call "brown." She shows Tom an advertisement for Florida orange juice and a traffic cone to demonstrate "orange"; UPS trucks and tree trunks to demonstrate "brown." But Tom just feels basketballs are more like tree trunks than traffic cones. Tom points out that basketballs are much less orange than Florida oranges, and that basketballs are the same color as his parents' new carpet which is called "rustic brown." Ann gets frustrated and finally begs Tom, "But don't you see it's orange?" Tom, equally frustrated, asks, "But don't you see it's brown?"

5. Cindy, a creationist and Bill, an atheist biologist, are having a debate about the origins of life. Bill says, "I have presented you with thousands of scientific articles, volumes of rational explanations, mountains of archaeological, geological, and biological evidence. Are you convinced of evolution now?" Cindy responds, "With all due respect, these types of evidence are not worth very much as evidence to me. No matter how many 'facts' or how much 'evidence' you show me, the most important evidence is 'the Word' revealed through the Holy Bible." Bill protests, "But I don't accept the Bible as fact." Cindy replies, "Well I don't accept scientific fact as fact." Bill says, "But science proves that science is the best evidence and contains the truth." Cindy says, "The Bible teaches that 'scientific evidence' can be illusion, and that the Bible contains the truth."
6. Rita speaks with her therapist, Frank. Frank explains, "Rita, you have been doing some unusual things: shouting in movie theaters, dressing strangely, crying at inappropriate times. We will work together to get your behavior back to normal." Rita asks, "Why should I want to be normal?" Frank says, "Normal is better than abnormal." Rita asks, "What exactly is better about it?" Frank explains, "Normal is more acceptable, less disturbing, less troubling to you and others, less bizarre." Rita responds, "What's so great about those things? What's so bad about being unacceptable, disturbing, troubled, and bizarre? You just want me to be normal because it's more normal." Frank says, "No, the value of being normal is that it allows you to enjoy normal things, a job, a family, friends. You may believe you don't want those normal things, but that is because you are not thinking normally."

Please do not take any of these examples as condoning substance-abuse, criminal acts, or destructive behavior of any kind. We can still hold the position that some things and some actions are better than others, even if we admit that we are operating within a paradigm; this exercise merely helps us to know exactly what we mean when we do so.

The takeaway I'd like to leave you with is: Paradigms *work* for those within the paradigm. Paradigms allow them to function. We need and use paradigms all the time to make progress.

Critical thinking can seem to halt the progress made by paradigms by stopping to ask hard questions about the paradigm itself, so if you wish to embark on a project of critical thinking, be aware that it may feel like you are holding up progress, that you are interfering with work, or that you are dys-functioning in any of several senses. Dealing with and overcoming this kind of resistance are part of the work of critical thinking.

9 Critical Thinking as a Set of Capacities

Critical thinking is about something subtler and, often, more important than getting results and solving problems. It is about awakening internal *capacities*, which includes making contact with ourselves and engaging with the world in an authentic way.

Treating critical thinking as a set of capacities should *substantially alter* how we conceive of teaching, facilitation, training, and coursework in critical thought. It should substantially shift our goals in these settings and it should shift how teachers and learners relate and interact therein. For instance, critical thinking leads us *to question* the meaning of the answers and to discover problems within the problems given to us, rather than merely solving them. That means that, when we are engaged with our critical thinking capacities, we often find that we have *more questions* at the end of a lesson or course than we did at the outset. We may see more problems and puzzles than we once did and we may even be more confused than we had been before.

We could reject critical thinking on this score, but while it may seem that critical thinking is only making our world more confusing, confusion is the first step in a longer process by which critical thinking makes our experience of ourselves and the world richer, more complex, and more profound.

Seeing things on their surfaces is easy, but critical thinking exposes us to a world of depth, complexity, and possibility we may have never otherwise considered. In other words, if we wish to pursue critical thinking, we must be prepared to experience some of the discomforts associated with ambiguity, doubt, and uncertainty.

The gamble implicit in this endeavor is that, in spite of the discomfort, what we will ultimately gain is a richer relationship with ourselves, with others, and with the world, a relationship in which we are both *freer* and more grounded than we were before because we are less influenced by "givens": prejudices, superficial knowledge, conventional wisdom, and the influence of norms, customs, habits, and unexamined assumptions.

Instead, if we have succeeded, we can call upon the capacity for critical thinking to keep our subjective world *fresh and alive*. Critical thinking may involve certain abilities, but, ultimately, if it is to connect to the individual's

DOI: 10.4324/9781003626398-11

subjectivity and his, her, or their true *being* in the world, it must be conceived of as a set of internal (intellectual, emotional, and psychological) *capacities* and, what is more, as a set of capacities whose exercise or dormancy is the very thing most worthy of study.

As I have alluded to above, what is set out in this part of this book is *not* a prescription for how to think critically. To organize a text in that way would, of course, be contrary to the very nature of the *facilitative* process – the process of allowing subjects to question, reflect, discover, and create new questions and answers – and would impinge upon the possibilities of critical thought, exploration, and discovery.

The most common error in teaching and learning critical thinking – and this applies not only to university or school life but also to professional trainings, career-building efforts, development projects, and more – is to imagine critical thinking to be a "skill" or "skill-set." To think of critical thinking as a skill or set of skills makes it like a *tool* or set of tools. This tool or set of tools, we believe, is something we can acquire and store in our cognitive "toolbox," ready to be called upon, at any moment, to solve problems.

The problem with conceiving of critical thinking in terms of skills or tools is that doing so makes critical thinking into a kind of static *object* we have at our disposal. When we think about critical thinking in this way, it becomes lifeless, and we, too, become lifeless in our pursuit and application of it.

We may come to think that once we have "acquired" this skill or tool, we need not attend to it ever again, that it will remain ready at hand in our "skill set" or "toolbox." Our attention is thus drawn away from the dynamic internal processes involved with critical thinking and, indeed, with the development of subjectivity. Our attention is drawn away from the need to attend to ourselves as subjects regularly in order to keep our ability to think alive. And our attention is drawn away from the fact that critical thinking is not exercised in a vacuum: There are scenarios, internal and external states, events, and environments that make critical thinking more and less difficult.

This error is likely to be familiar to those who were educated in the United States in the last half-century. Here, we have focused so intently on instruments of assessment, "objective" results, and measurable "outcomes," that schooling has come to mean little more than getting a sufficient quantity of correct answers to move on to the next level of schooling. We have focused on tests, numbers, and quantifiable results to such a degree that most students will tell you that their educations have infrequently engaged their internal processes of thought and emotion, their true capacities for critical thought and refection, and, therefore, their own subjective development.

What Is a Capacity?

A capacity is an internal state that can be brought to life. Capacities are things we do (or can do) that are connected to our *being*, which is to say: We can only activate our mental capacities to the extent that we exist psychically, to the extent that we are real, alive, and present.

Unlike the usual understandings of "skills" or "tools," capacities change, grow, and diminish over time. Capacities need to be exercised in order to remain available, like muscles, which is another way of saying that if we neglect to exercise a capacity we have developed, over time that capacity will become more difficult to access, mobilize, or realize in our selves and in the world.

What is nice about the term "capacity" is that it also refers us to the related term, "capacious," which alludes to, among other things, the availability of both space and power. The use of the term "capacity," then, suggests two important things about critical thinking.

1. The language of "capacity" is helpful insofar as we regard mental (intellectual, emotional, and psychological) development not as a linear process, where one stage is supplanted by another, but as a process of *multi-dimensional expansion*, where various parts of self increase or decrease in size, shape, prominence, and the like.

To develop one capacity does not necessarily mean to cover over another, nor to eliminate entirely what might stand in the way of its exercise from the psyche. Capacities develop or de-develop according to a variety of factors, perhaps the most important of which are:

- the foundation and early facilitation of the capacity,
- the security with which the capacity lives and is established in the inner world,
- the exercise or neglect of the capacity over time,
- the "internal objects" (i.e., internal psychological figures and forces) that are associated with it and surround it, and
- the "external objects" (i.e., external figures and forces) that influence, liberate, welcome, threaten, or otherwise exert pressure on the capacity.

If the capacity to think for ourselves is poorly or weakly facilitated in life, if it is constantly threatened or hardly ever exercised, or if internal objects in our psyches regularly attack it and make us feel guilt or shame for thinking for ourselves, then we are likely to have a tenuous hold on this capacity and are unlikely to be able to activate or make use of it.

On the contrary, if the capacity is founded in a facilitative process both early in life and later, throughout the course of life, if the exercise of the capacity does not feel dangerous, and if the capacity is exercised regularly, then this capacity will be relatively well established, secure, and we will be able to be call upon and act upon it.

2. The language of "capacity" suggests that we have to "make room" somewhere inside ourselves if we wish to develop new capacities. Ironically, we can become so busy and preoccupied with life that we neglect to make any room, inside ourselves, *for our selves*.

The feeling associated with this lack of room or space for the self is typically one of depression, dormancy, or lifelessness, or anxiety, futility, or emptiness – since we have nowhere *to be*.

Without a place *to be* inside ourselves, we may feel that we are being squeezed or pressed from all sides. It is, in any case, not a state in which we can engage in critical thinking because *the doer* who *does* the critical thinking *has no space* to think, to feel, to question, to be puzzled, or to act.

Not only do we have to make time in our lives to devote to critical thinking, we have to *open ourselves* to what we may learn or discover in the process in such a way that we "make room" for these things to connect with something inside us, in our inner worlds.

10 Resilience and Growing-up Experience

Critical Thinking and Resilience

So far, I have argued that critical thinking ought to be understood as a set of internal capacities. One important reason for doing so, not yet explored in depth, is that approaching critical thinking as such helps us to see its connection with *resilience* against pressures and powers, arising from within and without, that shut us down or do the opposite of critical thinking.

By "the opposite of critical thinking," I mean *not* thinking but, instead, conforming, obeying, adapting, suppressing oneself, or submerging one's intellectual and emotional existence into a corporation, family, nation, university, or any other group, real or imagined.

It is difficult to say whether a book on critical thinking is enough to alter the course of the life of a young adult who is otherwise subjected only to instruction, authority, and demands for obedience and conformity, as there are many forces far more powerful than a book, both in the early life of the family and later, in professional, civic, and social life, that exert tremendous influence.

Nevertheless, if teachers and significant others can help facilitate opportunities for learners to work on critical thinking, then learners will have that much more *resilience* in the face of the manifold powers and pressures that thwart its exercise.

For instance, in Stanley Milgram's famous *Obedience* experiments, participants were made to believe that they were doing real harm to other human beings.[1] Standing outside of the pressures of the situation, and looking at it in retrospect, it is easy to say that we would have thought more critically than they and would have known the right thing to do.

But that is precisely the point: These persons, many of whom were intelligent, thoughtful, and kind, failed to exercise critical thinking precisely because the situation in which they found themselves overwhelmed their capacities for critical thinking. Their capacities for critical thinking were not sufficiently *resilient* to withstand the forces that told them to de-activate their thinking, to refuse to consider the situation, or to judge their actions thoughtfully. Rather,

DOI: 10.4324/9781003626398-12

they behaved in ways that others demanded, rather than in ways that expressed who they truly were.

The ease with which we fulfill scripted roles and obey authorities tells us something about our psychic landscapes: that they are not places where critical thought, creativity, reason, and autonomous judgment reign *alone*, but, rather, where internalized images of others, unconscious fantasies, and susceptibilities to compliance, conformity, and adaptation the needs or expectations of others are ready to obstruct our ability to think critically, even when we seem to be "free" to do so.

Christopher Bollas has famously suggested the category of the "unthought known" to describe that which is never cognitively processed but nevertheless becomes a person's basic orientation to self and to life.[2] Bollas' argument is that, at the level of inner experience, we may "know" something without ever "thinking" about it. It may be incorporated so completely in our basic intellectual and emotional frameworks that it can only be repeated and repeated again throughout our lives.

To imagine that an individual can simply apply learned methods or behaviors in order to "think" about his or her "unthought known" would be to seriously underestimate the difficulty and complexity of this task. And yet, this is a significant part of the task of critical thinking, such that we may even say that critical thinking must inevitably address "the unthought known" as one of its primary targets.

Critical Thinking and Growing-Up Experiences

The degree to which we comply and the degree to which we resist – in favor of autonomy and creativity – depends in an important way on our early *growing-up experiences*, in which, as children, we were subjected to the demands of others, and, most importantly, of caregivers on whom we depended and whom we loved. I will offer an unusual glimpse into some of my own growing-up experiences and my attempts to bring critical thinking to them in the lengthy penultimate chapter, Chapter 15.

The timing, setting, and manner in which demands were issued, the way we, as children, interpreted them, the consequences that followed or seemed to follow from questioning or failing to satisfy them, and the emotional toll these complex experiences took on us, as children, formed the foundation (or lack thereof) on which the capacity for critical thought could later be built.

In many cases – and I do not wish to draw too dire of a picture here – obedience and compliance is *all* a child can do, since he, she, or they rarely possess the wherewithal, the mental capacities, or the physical presence or strength to "resist" the pressure of demands of parents, teachers, and other adults.

Worse: These demands are often couched in language and relationships that are complex and confusing, such that a parent may ask a child to do something that the child hates, that the child would never willingly do, or that the child finds terrible or terrifying, but the demand may be framed as a compliment about the child's independence and courage, or the child's willingness to be "big" or responsible. This linking of terror and praise, hatred and independence, can become quite confounding for a child, and, indeed, for many adults, who often need help in untying the psychological "knots" by which they have long felt tied.

Even worse: There are many instances in which the child's failure to comply with the demands of caregivers or authorities seems to the child to be extremely dangerous. (And, indeed, a failure to comply may very well be dangerous, at either a physical level or a psychic level of experience.) If a choice is presented to a child thus: "Obey me or lose my love and protection," virtually all children will obey, not only because the child physically depends on the care and protection of the caregiver, but because, emotionally, the demand *itself* places the child in a horrifying world where being loved (and being worthy of love), protected, and kept alive are no longer things that can be counted on reliably, but are *conditional upon not thinking or being himself, herself, or themselves,* i.e., upon being an object and not a subject, on carrying out obedient and self-effacing behavior.

Should the child's behavior fail to please the caregiver, then the child may be thrown into a world of unimaginable anxiety, loss, deprivation, and terror: a world without love or safety. This turns the child's inner world into a place where survival (not just physical but emotional survival) is always in doubt and, thus, where subjectivity is a luxury that simply cannot be afforded.

It is vitally important that the environment in which critical thinking is undertaken *not* replicate or reinforce the dilemmas in which the child (now the aspiring subject) feels forced to obey at risk of losing love, attention, care, or support. At the same time, teachers and facilitators of critical thinking must recognize that they cannot expect students to be ready and willing to undertake the work of questioning paradigms, challenging tradition and authority, stepping outside the safety of the group, and the like, without doing considerable psychological work to assure that the environment in which nascent subjects find themselves is a "new" one, one that is *not* the environment of the family or the authority-led group, but, rather, an open and democratic space that is, itself, *capacious* enough to welcome the free exercise of the students' capacities for critical thinking.

Notes

1 Stanley Milgram, *Obedience to Authority: An Experimental View* (New York: Harper & Row, 1974).

2 Christopher Bollas, *The Shadow of the Object: Psychoanalysis of the Unthought Known* (New York: Columbia University Press, 1987), 277–83.

11 The Dilemma of Activation

One considerable obstacle to critical thinking – what I have come to think of as a very specific problem – is what I call the *dilemma of activation*. The dilemma of activation describes the situation in which a person has the opportunity to think critically about a choice, an idea, or a decision, and to use critical thinking to inform his, her, or their judgment or action, but *does not recognize* that the time, place, or problem is one in which critical thinking is called for.

The relationship between critical thinking and judgment is complex, but even more complex perhaps is the fact that, in order to bring one's capacities for critical thinking to a matter, one must *first* – somehow – judge that the matter is appropriate for, suitable for, and worthy of critical thinking.

There is an ancient paradox about learning that parallels this dilemma, articulated best by Aristotle, who recognized that if one were truly ignorant – as we all are in certain respects and on certain issues – then one would not be aware that there was anything more one needed to know. Thus, one would be unlikely to seek learning and, worse, one would not know what learning or knowledge one needed.

The problem of activation is similar, in that, first, one must judge a situation to be amenable or appropriate for critical thinking, then, second, do the work of critical thinking. But how can one critically judge whether to think critically if one has not already activated one's capacities for critical thinking?

That is, how does one critically think about *whether* to think critically?

One way to resolve this dilemma – but not a sensible way – is to maintain that we should *always* use our capacity for critical thinking. But this is a rather foolish notion, if we consider it carefully. We cannot think critically about everything, all the time. We must, in many situations of daily life, rely on habit, on "given" knowledge, and on reasonably held beliefs taken on the authority of others. For example, we do not question and re-question the law of gravity at every instant, grasping at the banister for fear of floating off into space. If we did, we would – perhaps literally – never get anywhere.

Likewise, we do not typically question whether a STOP sign really means to stop, or, rather, expresses a different command in an unknown language, or has

DOI: 10.4324/9781003626398-13

been planted there by mischievous vandals, or is a hallucination. Most of the time, for our own safety and that of others, we just stop the car.

And most of us believe, reasonably, I think, that the planets in our solar system have certain properties and features, such as rings, moons, and the like, solely on the authority of astronomers, even though we may never have studied these planets for ourselves nor observed their features through telescopes or with our own eyes.

A different, but equally facile and uninformed, manner of resolving the dilemma of activation is to argue that is *easy* to know when we to activate our capacity for critical thinking. For instance, if we sit on a jury weighing evidence in a criminal case, the judge will repeatedly issue direct orders to all jurors to think carefully about the evidence at hand, to disregard bias and prejudice, and to adjudicate reasonably and fairly.

All this, plus the fact that a person's life may hang in the balance, tends to lead jurors, if not to think hard, at least to hear a call from within and without to activate their capacity for critical thinking, or so we should like to believe. Whether the jurors have developed the capacity for critical thinking, and to what extent they are able to bring that capacity to bear on the matter at hand – when faced with the influences of the attorneys and the other jurors and their own feelings and beliefs about the case, the accuser and the accused, the judge, and more – is another matter.

We may be tempted to believe that any time a human life is involved, we will be prompted to mobilize our capacity for critical thinking, owing to the gravity of the situation. Unfortunately, situations involving harm or potential harm to others *do not* always activate in us the judgment that we ought to bring critical thinking to bear on the situation. In fact, they often do the opposite, by activating our defenses against accepting the full weight of that responsibility.

The gravity of such situations, the power and pressures embedded in the environments, the weight of all that is at stake, the need to be "right" – which may come to mean: the need to have one's judgment and conduct affirmed by an authority or group – and the unconscious pull to fulfill roles in a moral drama are more than often enough to utterly deactivate or suppress our capacities for critical thought.

In the Nazi Holocaust, many victimizers' capacities for critical thinking were foreclosed or de-activated by the power and pressures of authority- and conformity-laden groups and settings. Indeed, both victims and victimizers unwittingly found themselves playing scripted roles in atrocious dramas that were not of their own making.[1]

Here, again, we may see why conceiving of critical thinking as a "skill" or "tool," always ready-at-hand, is an impoverished notion. Many persons possess the cognitive abilities to make logical inferences and deductions. Yet, what is lacking in those who fail to use critical thinking when they should is not merely proficiency in reasoning or thinking "skills," but, rather, a special sort of *resilient insight* that permits both the activation of and the exercise of the relevant capacities in an environment where critical thinking seems unwelcome.

That last one was a complex sentence, so let me put it another way: Often, what persons who fail to call upon critical thinking *lack* is the ability to resist – to hold at bay – the pressures applied to them, to stop and wonder whether this or that moment would be a good time to call upon their critical thinking capacities, and to determine whether to question, problematize, or reflect further upon what they must judge or do. So, they fail to recognize the situation as one in which critical thinking is called for, even when it seems obvious to us, or to others outside, or in the eyes of history, that the situation is just that.

There is no perfect resolution to the dilemma of activation. The best we can do is to hope that, if a person has developed the capacities for critical thinking and has become more of a subject than an object, then he, she, or they are more likely to have established a channel of communication with himself, herself, or themselves, which, in turn, makes him, her, or them more likely to experience an oppressive situation as oppressive, as a situation that is impinging upon abilities to think, to judge, to reason.

Ideally, such impingement would send up a kind of warning signal to the individual (this signal may be anxiety or a feeling of confinement, or any number of things, depending on the individual) that he, she, or they have entered into a complex situation, where powerful forces are at work and, thus, that require attention, reflection, and critical thought.

Note

1 For a detailed and compelling study of these events as seen through the eyes of "ordinary men" recruited to conduct exterminations in Poland, see Christopher R. Browning, *Ordinary Men: Reserve Police Battalion 101 and the Final Solution in Poland* (New York: HarperCollins, 1992).

12 The Dilemma of Teaching and the Solution of Facilitation

Related to the dilemma of activation, there is an apparent paradox at the heart of the endeavor of teaching critical thinking. It is the same apparent paradox that appears in the teaching of many subjects, in the practice of psychology, in parenting, in ministries of various kinds, and in a host of other familial, social, cultural, and political activities.

The apparent paradox is this:

On one hand: critical thinking means thinking freely and autonomously, with minimal interference from given or predetermined beliefs and from the influence of others.

On the other hand: The teaching of critical thinking usually requires that learners follow a guided course of study, that they be given assignments, exercises, and tasks (pre)determined by the teacher(s), and even that they be receptive to the suggestions, instructions, and influence of the teacher(s).

The paradox, however, is merely an apparent one (i.e., not a *true* paradox) if we consider the process of *facilitation*, whose ideal is to make the discovery of the capacity for critical thinking available and attainable for the learner.

Facilitation is a method of teaching and learning, the method most reasonable to employ in the teaching of critical thinking if one conceives critical thinking to be a set of capacities related to the development of the subjecthood of learners. If this is our understanding and our goal, any other method of teaching critical thinking would transform the apparent paradox into a true, and tragic, paradox.

Facilitation means, first, opening up space for learners to question, explore, discover, and create ideas in ways that rely on and build up their capacities to think freely and autonomously.

Facilitation accomplishes this by introducing problems, frameworks, puzzles, and possibilities *without* determining too much, without imposing final answers.

Facilitation encourages the learner to generate and ask his, her, or their own questions, as I have argued in a popular article in the National

DOI: 10.4324/9781003626398-14

Education Association Journal *Thought & Action*, to make self-discovery on the part of the learner important parts (indeed, fundamental parts) of the learning-process.[1]

§

I use the term "facilitate" in its most robust sense. The facilitation of intellectual processes related to critical thinking is not passive, hands-off, or *laissez-faire*, or at least it is not necessarily so. Facilitation may include periods of direct instruction, of listening, of challenging, and more.

What is key about facilitation is that when one facilitates, one facilitates the growth of the capacities of another, in this case, the capacities of the learner. The ideal of facilitation emphasizes the way that the learner's development – particularly in critical thinking – is related to the discovery of capacities and potentialities within the learner, fostered by an appropriate learning environment. The antitheses of facilitation are *neglect* or *impingement*, which involve, respectively, abandonment-induced deprivation, on one hand, and the imposition and disruption of critical thinking activities by external forces, on the other.

The same holds true in the other endeavors mentioned above. A responsible minister, for example, neither neglects to care for parishioners nor dictates to parishioners what to think or to believe. The minister does neither simply gives them rules to follow, nor strives to influence parishioners to believe exactly what the minister believes. Rather, the minister *facilitates* in parishioners *their own capacities* to make meaningful contact with the special part of themselves to which the work of ministry attends.

Similarly, a thoughtful psychologist does not simply drop patients into emotional freefall, nor inform patients precisely how to feel and behave, but, rather, facilitates a process by which patients arrive, by their own efforts, at a better understanding of themselves. In this way, patients both discover something valuable and "own" what is discovered: the capacities for critical thinking, self-reflection, self-discovery, personality-integration, change, and development.

Parenting, where the ultimate goal is to facilitate the capacities in the child that will allow the child to thrive in the adult world, if not handled properly, can thwart the facilitation of maturation and replace it with embeddedness in a power relationship, based on either fear of abandonment or dependence on authority. The result of such a failure of parenting may well be that a child comes to live in an adult's body.

The child-adult may always or often behave "properly," but may not know who he, she, or they *really are*, why he, she, or they behave in certain ways, or what he, she, or they really think or feel. In this way, the child in the body of an adult can only conform to what has been given to or determined by the surroundings, lacking the capacity to do the work of critical thinking, to reason, to judge, or to act in meaningful ways, ways that express his, her, or their subjectivity and genuine presence in the world.

Note

1 Matthew H. Bowker, "Teaching Students to Ask Questions Instead of Answering Them," *Thought and Action: The NEA Higher Education Journal* 26, no. 1 (2010): 127–34.

Part III

Lessons in Subject-Activation

Honesty, Patience, and Bravery

13 Living and (Almost) Dying Honestly

Even if we've done a lot of work with critical thinking, most of us can still recall, identify with, or even feel the experience of being a child in an adult's body. It is unpleasant, to say the least. It generally feels like powerlessness, hopelessness, or emptiness. It can lead us to believe there is something wrong with us, that we do not pass muster, or that we are not qualified to live. It can involve thinking that our very selves are unreal and therefore nonexistent, evanescent, ephemeral. It can bring with it un-creativity, boring compliance, and inner deadness.

On the other hand, one of the surest ways to come alive as a subject, to take up a more grounded and free position as a mature subject is to undertake an honest self-appraisal, applying critical thought to oneself.

This honest critical approach to the self can feel embarrassing, shameful, even terrifying, since we compare our own truths to the mythical truths of the great machinery, and are worried we might find ourselves coming up short. Thus, we can feel most like a lost child at the very moments when our true *subjective being* is actually starting to break through.

This first chapter of this section of the book is devoted to an example of dysfunction, honesty, and maturation into a subjective state. It's a story of an escapade I undertook many years ago.

§

After college, I dysfunctioned. Actually, I had already dysfunctioned by spending my senior year not in residence at my home university but in Paris studying abroad. My friends stayed behind, polished their resumes, and got interviews for high-paying jobs after graduation. I wanted to go to Paris and then to West Africa, caring little for the path of getting a "good job" back in the U.S.A. After graduating *in absentia*, I flew off to Porto-Novo, Benin, a representative country of the region.

I had no arrangements when I landed in Benin other than a piece of paper with a man's name on it: Lucien, who lived in Porto-Novo and was said to run a farm nearby. I was sick from the travel but eventually made it to the capital city and asked around until I found Lucien. I inquired if I could work on his farm

DOI: 10.4324/9781003626398-16

but was told that the farm was no longer operational. Rather, Lucien had started a small, local enterprise, currently in the business of collecting garbage around the city. I was offered a place to sleep (semi-outdoors) and a giant sack of corn meal in exchange for my labor pushing one of the enormous, green, covered wheelbarrows called "*charettes*," used to collect garbage by hand.

Let me say a few things about this experience. Porto-Novo, while indeed the capital city, is very little like a city by Western standards. It is not a highly developed urban area. "Roads" meant dirt paths. There was no electricity, there were no streetlights, there were no grocery stores or hospitals. In the area where I lived, water to drink or to wash came from wells or, if you were lucky, out of a shared pump that supposedly hooked up with a clean source. My meals were, by and large, boiled cornmeal, shared and eaten by hand. My "bed" was a collection of half a dozen disused, small "*pupitres*" (small chairs connected to small desks). The "garbage" we collected consisted primarily of human feces, dumped in piles by the majority of residents without toilets or sewers. I, too, had no toilet or sewer system and, for my time there, made use of a deep hole behind a sort of shack used primarily to offer shade from the sun.

In spite of, or because of, all of these difficulties, I worked hard and connected with myself in a special way in the months I lived there. I had undertaken this mission because of a personal, inner impulse. I wanted to see what life in a truly underdeveloped area was like. I wanted to live it, to see if I could learn something useful (for myself and for others) from the experience. I critically examined this impulse before, during, and after my trip. I felt close to it, ultimately to find that my own mature subjectivity was deeply interwoven with it.

While in Benin, my critical thinking efforts revolved around a handful of notepads for journaling and only two small books I threw in my rucksack upon leaving: *Jitterbug Perfume*, a humorous novel by Tom Robbins, and a pocket edition of the *Dao De Jing*.[1] *Jitterbug Perfume* will forever remain a part of my mental life because, beyond the humor and casualness of Robbins' style, there I found characters who were deeply in touch with their own subjective impulses and desires. The *Dao De Jing* was, obviously, quite different, but reading it in Africa, in "nature," and in a place where I had to assert myself regularly against the elements brought me close to it in a way I had not expected. Almost 30 years later, with many re-visitations in between, I finally felt ready to compose a translation of it.[2]

In the notepads I kept daily journals in which I mostly interrogated myself about my thoughts and feelings.

- *What did I want?*
- *What did I need?*
- *What was I really doing there?*
- *Why and where did I feel pain and sadness?*
- *How would I make meaning in my life when my trip was over?*

These journals became so intimate to me I would have fought to the death if someone had tried to take them away.

A funny thing happens when you interrogate yourself daily and on paper: You become honest. Or at least, I became honest. I told myself that I had to write with utter honesty and integrity, including about deeply difficult things, in order to develop the kind of relationship with myself that I wanted as an adult.

In turn, this lesson taught me that, in my project of critically coming to know myself, I had to be honest not just in my writing but in everything I said and did. I decided in Africa that, no matter what, I would be honest with myself and others, I would never renege on an obligation (because I would not say "I will" to something I could not or would not do), I would keep all promises, even and especially to myself, and my personal journey would be full of honest self-conversation about my emotions, ideas, achievements, and defeats. I would confront myself, face to face, with both my demons and my highest ideals, and I would think about them critically to see what I could learn, to discover who I was, and to see who I would become.

The garbage-collecting work was brutal and the heat was brutal and, to some extent, the self-work in my journals was a bit more brutal than it had to be. In any case, after several months, perhaps from infection, exhaustion, or both, I became gravely ill. I could not eat. I could barely move. I could only sleep, and I slept, without eating or moving, for over a week. I looked emaciated. Occasionally, people came by to look in on me and I would pry open my eyes to see someone standing over me, saying something in Fon about how I may not get better or how it was likely malaria. There was no talk of doctors or medicine or hospitals and, to be frank, I was young enough and naïve enough not to think of them either. One morning, I recall hearing my friend praying for me outside my ramshackle hut at dawn.

I remember believing that I was, almost assuredly, going to die. Instead of panicking, however, I felt a strange sense of comfort and serenity. I thought of everything I had learned from my critical thinking work and how close I had become with myself. I had come to love my self, although in a non-narcissistic way. What I mean is: I had developed a loving attitude toward the person I was, the person I had become. It took some work, to be sure, for me to learn to love myself. I don't think I had ever loved myself before. The main ingredient, the primary difference, was my honest work in critical thinking.

Obviously, to be honest is helpful if one wishes to avoid cheating, stealing, and lying. But more to the point, you can't do critical thinking work without being honest with yourself. If you can be honest with yourself, you won't hide behind façades or false fronts because your *critical thinking capacities* will go to work unmasking the fraud. You won't make excuses for yourself or others: Your *critical* mind will see right through them.

At the same time, if you can be honest with yourself, you realize that you have to be *creative*, in the sense that you have to wake up and *create* a new, authentic self every day. You have to choose the standard that your day is going to meet. You won't take on more than you can handle. And when you do take on a lot, since you have to be honest, you'll find that you have no choice but to rise to the challenge and finish what you started.

One of the best parts of doing critical thinking work is that, if you are honest, you can't help but recognize that all human beings are frail and fallible. This realization allowed me to escape from a good deal of self-imposed *guilt and shame*, since, ultimately, every person is in the same boat, all doing our best, all deserving of love and forgiveness, and I was one of those frail, fallible persons.

Some inner calling had led me to travel to a deeply underdeveloped city in Africa and to work as a garbage collector. In following that impulse, and in continuing to follow the path of honest critical thought, my mature, subjective presence and personality began to come to life, and for this I was, above all, grateful.

Needless to say, I did not die. It took some weeks, but I recovered my strength. I left Africa soon after that, although I had planned to stay longer, because I felt I had learned the most important lesson there was to learn: Subjectivity thrives on honesty, making honest critical thinking the very core of living a life of integrity, depth, and meaning. It shaped how I navigated external challenges then, but also how I cultivated more meaningful, forgiving, and loving relationships with myself and others. Honesty allowed me to trust myself, to set realistic boundaries, and to rise to challenges when necessary. Honesty led to groundedness and freedom, the groundedness and freedom that come from subjective being.

§

I think it is important to slow down for a moment and clarify a few of the ideas just raised. I have spoken a lot about honesty, without ever really defining it. What do we mean when we say "honesty"? I have come to think of honesty in less strict, you might say less "Western" and less rationalistic terms. I no longer think of it just as a *law* one makes for oneself. Now I think of honesty in relation to subjectivity, genuineness, spontaneity, authenticity, and even creativity. It may seem strange to speak of it this way.

I like to think I learned some things from the copy of the *Dao De Jing* I brought with me on my travels, so it seems appropriate to take an example from Daoist teachings, which are very often simple allegories about nature. Why don't we start by saying that a mountain stream flows *honestly*. If it is pristine, it moves and turns and runs and falls in a way that we are tempted to call *genuine* and *unique* to the stream. Indeed, we may even say the stream is forever *authentic* and *spontaneous*, not "spontaneous" in the sense of "sudden" or "momentary," but in the broader sense of "self-directing." A *spontaneous* gesture is not guided by others' plans, coaxed by ulterior aims or ends, or shaped by external pressures. Instead, it *comes from somewhere inside* the thing itself, from its being, and *expresses itself for its own sake*.

The water in the stream gushes down the mountain, according to its own natural path. Again, this is not to say that the stream is unaffected by its surroundings: the rocks and the soil and the trees and the rainfall all exert an influence. But the stream *flows* because the stream *is* and the stream's *being* is reflected in its *doing*. If we were to intervene and block the stream and divert it for some other purpose, we could say we would be interfering with its honest path, its true, natural flow.

The *Dao* simply means "the way." It is not something that the creators of Daoism, like Laozi or Zhuangzi, imagined could be put into words. To try to force it into words would be a kind of insult, they thought. Rather, the Dao was generally thought of as a power (which is not *forceful*) that is creative, spontaneous, and self-generating. We cannot name it not primarily because it is too big or sublime to be named. Rather, we cannot name it because, once we name it, it becomes a standardized way, a road already traveled by. The early philosophers of the Dao wanted to reserve it for "the way" that has not developed into anything rote or standardized, like a practice. Although undefinable, the Dao has certain identifiable characteristics, such as: simplicity, effortlessness, authenticity, harmony, and nonattachment.

Honesty, in this sense, means living in accordance with the principles that guide the Dao, particularly, I would say, in inner life. Honesty is a form of integrity. The stream has its integrity (i.e., it remains a stream) so long as it is not dammed up, diverted into three or four alternate paths, collected, pooled, and so on. Likewise, we have *integrity* (a loaded word, I know) in our inner lives to the extent that we feel as if we are connected to the truths inside us, not split off from them, not diverted or distracted from them.

I want to say: *Being* is not *true being* if it is not *honest*. Thus, honest critical thinking is needed for honest *being*. The very idea of *being*, in philosophy as in psychoanalysis, suggests that authenticity works as a modifier, whereas falsehood characterizes one of being's alternatives, such as *seeming*. *Being* requires honesty. *Seeming* relies on dissemblance.

§

Psychologically speaking, we have to *be* before we can *do* anything really genuine. We have to try to make sure that our *doing* arises out of our *being*, or else we may undertake doing that arises from a false self, which, of course, is a way of *seeming* but not *being*.

Donald Winnicott argued that many moments of our lives, especially if we are not thoughtful, are taken up with activity that is nonauthentic, and this kind of activity he understood as the *doing* that expresses *not being*. Winnicott believed that the basis of authentic being was creativity. We have to have some creative center, some experience of ourselves as really and truly alive in order to *be*. From this position of deep, inner motility we can learn to *be creative* out into the world.[3] As infants, if we were given the opportunity by our parents, we imagined we created the whole world, insofar as we imagined our very *being* made everything happen. We have touched on some of these ideas briefly in Chapter 5.

Winnicott believed that one of the most important caregiving functions of a parent was to "hold" the infant emotionally by taking care of its needs and by responding to its impulses with great sensitivity. "Holding" means neither squeezing nor dropping the infant, but, rather, helping the infant to remain in a kind of suspended animation where it is not even aware that it is being held. In a "holding environment," wishes come true and infants "create the world." The infant wishes for milk and, before it is even fully aware of this wish, milk appears. (In reality, the parent provides milk at the appropriate time.) In a holding environment, the infant smiles and, without having to try or to ask, a parent appears to mirror the child by smiling right back.[4]

The "holding" (and later, "handling") environment sets the stage for the infant's authentic being to emerge. Holding provides a safe space where the infant feels able to explore, play, and act spontaneously, authentically, and creatively on its innermost impulses. That is, through the attunement of the parents to the infant, the infant is granted the ability to experience its own authentic being in reality.

The reality of the infant in this situation is naturally abundant, simple, fluid, and supported. The infant exists in a kind of "flow state" which Winnicott termed "going on being."[5] "Going on being" means exactly what it sounds like. In a healthy environment, the infant will discover what we may call a continuity of experience. The infant flows from one operation to the next, weaves in and out of fantasy and reality, and feels itself the center of a universe with no limits.

Although no particular infant is, literally, the center of the universe, for a short period of time, every infant must experience itself to be the center of the universe if it is going to get on with the project of being and developing. As the center of all things, the infant effortlessly brings real and unreal objects into and out of existence, calls up and sends away what it likes or dislikes, feels into itself and out of itself in turn, and in general, lives and plays effortlessly.

If we were to make a kind of analogy: The effortlessness of nature for the Daoist is the magic of the holding environment for Winnicott. Daoist teachings suggest that we can live in a kind of balance with nature and with the Dao, which, I would like to suggest, is really another way of saying that we can regain a piece of our own simple, unadorned, and child-like nature. When individuals live in harmony with these natures, they feel supported and peaceful, just as infants find the holding environment to provide the requisite safety and containment for their true selves to come creatively alive in reality. The holding environment, like the Dao, offers a space where one feels safe and supported, allowing for the natural development of the self in an organic and unforced way. Both Winnicott's holding environment and the nature of the Dao provide the conditions for authenticity and psychological health.

Unfortunately, it is not long before temptations arise in the form of others whom we want or need to please. Once we lose attunement with that little kernel of ourselves that was truly authentic and genuine, focusing our attention instead on the reality of others whose expectations we have to meet, we lose our capacity to be creative, spontaneous, authentic, and free. We begin acting uncreatively, according to others' agendas or rules, for the sake of performance, for the pleasure of others, or to fit into some given or fixed image or ideal of who we are or must be. Once this happens, we are no longer acting honestly or creatively. We are reacting, obeying, or conforming. We are doing the doing that expresses our lack and loss of honest being.

Notes

1 Tom Robbins, *Jitterbug Perfume*. New York: Bantam Books, 1984; Lao Tzu, *Tao Te Ching*, trans. John C.H. Wu (Boston: Shambhala Publications, 1989).
2 M.H. Bowker, *The Dao De Jing: A Subversive Transcreation* (Unpublished Manuscript, likely publication date 2026).
3 D.W. Winnicott, *Home is Where We Start From: Essays by a Psychoanalyst*, eds. Clare Winnicott, Ray Shepherd, and Madeleine Davis (New York: W.W. Norton & Company, 1986).
4 D.W. Winnicott, "The Theory of the Parent-Infant Relationship," in *The Maturational Processes and the Facilitating Environment* (New York: International Universities Press, 1965), 37–55.
5 D.W. Winnicott, "Ego Integration in Child Development," in *The Maturational Processes and the Facilitating Environment* (New York: International Universities Press, 1965), 56–63.

14 Patience, Breaking, and Writing

Africa was a long time ago. Since then, I had known peace and I had lost it, time and again. I embarked on all sorts of new and different adventures, some less deliberately planned, and most not without disturbance. Yet, for the most part, I was free. To live honestly in the work of critical thinking does not mean that we are immune to pain and suffering. Indeed, sometimes, the honesty and clarity I have tried to describe above can make the reality of pain and suffering all the more acute, as we can't shut it out or numb ourselves to it.

Ever since I returned from Africa, I wanted to become a writer. I failed a lot at first. I didn't only fail to get published, I failed to write anything I thought was good enough to try to publish. Today, people are impressed by the fact that I have written about 20 books, in a variety of genres, on top of dozens of scholarly articles, chapters, and papers. What they don't know is that anything I write that is any good comes from a place of deep and honest being, a place I have found only by burrowing deeper and deeper than I thought possible to find the truth.

I had a friend from college who was very interested in writing spiritual, inspirational books. I think I learned, through his mistakes, what I needed to remember about critical thinking and the creative (subjective) process. My friend wanted very much to be enlightened and to find the kind of spiritual peace he found described in the writings and teachings he knew. But he really wanted this spiritual good to be part of his success, a prideful goal wherein others would recognize him as a leader, a teacher, a guru of sorts. He was, in essence, a depressed person who fantasized about getting validation from others as a way to escape his depression through achievement: *How could he be a guru and be depressed?* He couldn't, he thought. So becoming a guru would, therefore, cure him of his depression.[1]

Because of the conflation or confusion of his goals, he could never let go, never let himself go, but was always picking up the pieces and pulling himself together, to be ahead of the game, to rebound from defeat quickly, to take another step forward, never to be seen in a bad light. I always wanted to tell my friend to stop, to let himself go, to let himself fall into pieces. He reminded me of a saying, common among psychologists, that depressed people can't sleep (and generally can't relax) because they cannot let themselves drop into non-doing and non-being.

DOI: 10.4324/9781003626398-17

Depressed people have been so hurt by their depression, it has been so painful for them, that they avoid even the hint of it at all costs. And it seems to loom around every corner. They are afraid of its return. Thus, they lie in bed awake, fearing that it might overtake them in the darkness of the room or even in a dream. They cannot let the reins of their selves go and get back to playing and being creative in life, because the creative play might lead to a dark place. Indeed, the possibility that creative play may lead us to a dark place is part of what makes the play exciting. Real creative play can handle dark places. It can even shine little lights in them and make them less scary. But only for those who can tolerate the initial darkness.

My First Poem

The very first poem I published appeared in a small literary journal called *Superficial Flesh*, sadly no longer in print. It took me a long time to write it. Every word seemed to take me hours, days to get just perfect. I had to practice a lot of patience with it. But I loved the work of trying to make everything precise, so the patience wasn't of the painful sort.

The poem, itself, is whimsical, humorous, dark, probing, and genuine all at the same time. It pokes fun at post-modern philosophy and culture, insisting in its own way that we still had the same basic, human problems that we have always had. It suggests a few new ways to think about those problems. It is called "7 postmodern problems in no particular hierarchical occidental phallological order." Here it is.

7 postmodern problems
in no particular hierarchical occidental phallological order

1.

Mustn't we resist
centro-centrism,
that nasty habit
of seeing centers,
sacre coeur,
brazen face, money shot,
centrally,
or
does privileging
peripheries,
borderline, *outre-mer*, otherskin,
only fetishize
marginalia?

2.

How infinitely disappointed
is the one who googles:
You search for me now.

3.

Is it I who grow balder, paler, fatter each year like an ugly angel send children's paper lanterns smashing through the ice leave out cookies for the cops not the good ones unplug everything but the television watch crows peck empty plastic bags in perfect parking lots consider carefully the time to buy new shoes feel the metaphorical depression of subletters subletting to subletters until nobody answers the door?

4.

What have we taught the student who writes:
"Cannibals are like vegetarians in America:
it's just a way of life."?

5.

If sin
is habituation,
and adaptation
is hereditary sin,
to what blade
barrel
beast
body
plot
gaze
mass
shall we
cease
to be
accustomed?

6.

When words, once spoken, die
within our hearts, then
isn't every poet, *amant, philosophe*
a special type of murderer,
and every psychoanalyst Kevorkian?

7.

What if I sign
in soy vinegar ink,
and gracious lower case,
but just lie my ass off,
as if I were not unweaving old wool,
or bisecting imaginary angles,
or with cupped hands pleading piously?[2]

It's a little weird, I know. But it is real. It came from an experience of extreme thinking and waiting, knowing only the word before me and not the next one or the next one.

Waiting

It took me a bit of agitation to learn to wait for things to come from myself, by themselves, when they were ready, which is like a kind of active letting-go. One of my heroes, Friedrich Nietzsche, wisely said that "a thought comes when 'it' wishes, and not when 'I' wish."[3] It is true, I can tell you from long experience. On the other end of the ideological spectrum, another one of my heroes, Christian scholar and contemplative, Thomas Merton, a Trappist monk, vibrant thinker, and true lover of God, wrote in *The Climate of Monastic Prayer*:

> The true contemplative is not one who prepares his mind for a particular message that he wants or expects to hear, but is one who remains empty because he knows that he can never expect to anticipate the words that will transform his darkness into light. He does not even anticipate a special kind of transformation. He does not demand light instead of darkness. He waits on the Word of God in silence, and, when he is "answered," it is not so much by a word that bursts into his silence. It is by his silence itself, suddenly, inexplicably revealing itself to him as a word of great power, full of the voice of God.[4]

That's how I would describe my most creative works: waiting in silent, critical, creative contemplation until the silence itself becomes speech, the most honest speech there is.

This insight has passed beyond the walls of the monastery, once again, in the work of Donald Winnicott. One of Winnicott's key contributions to the psychoanalytic and clinical literatures was his insistence upon natural processes that took their own time. The proper stance, then, of the clinician was very often simply to wait.

"If we can adjust ourselves to these natural processes," he wrote, "we can leave most of these complex mechanisms to nature, while we sit back and watch and learn."[5] He quipped: "As a psychoanalyst, I have had very good training in this matter of waiting and waiting and waiting."[6]

In caring for patients, Winnicott suggested a nonintrusive clinical method, comparing what happened in the therapeutic setting to what happens, on a broader scale, in development, where people can only grow on their own time. Winnicott's method was minimalistic, regarding the resistance often encountered by patients as hesitations, rather than full blockages. Winnicott wished to give time to such hesitations, rather than to attack them, for the patient only comes to himself in his own time.[7]

I think this is how we ought to treat ourselves: with patience. We can feel a sense of urgency in undertaking the work of honest critical thinking and subjective becoming. But so often, we find ourselves rushed to attain and achieve that we skip that work and end up feeling lost. So often we find ourselves intolerant of things in our lives or parts of ourselves that seem to get in the way. We can be really ruthless toward ourselves, more brutal than a therapist would ever be to a patient. Instead, we should let ourselves be. We should *even let ourselves be broken*, and then wait to see what happens as we naturally and slowly heal, even if we heal crookedly.

Everything I have written since that first poem has come out of a place of paradoxical brokenness *and* wholeness, the wholeness that comes from accepting, inviting, and then plumbing the brokenness. Once broken, we are no longer tethered to the course we were on when we were of a piece, forced together. Now, we can do anything.

§

I want to tell you about two tattoos. I got them at roughly the same time, the first while teaching courses in Singapore, the second shortly after my return. They were two discoveries that I wanted to remember. The first says "I can do anything" in Mandarin. Warned against having too much "ego," there was some discussion among the tattoo artists of whether or not I should keep the 我, the Chinese character for "I." Without it, an adjusted phrase could read more like: "Anything is possible." That is not what I wanted.

At the risk of being *ego*tistical or a "biggo," as the Singaporeans called it, I wanted to remind myself that I was both free enough and capable enough to do whatever I wanted. That seems like a narcissistic fantasy, I know, but I meant it with humility. I had, by that time, earned a Ph.D., become accomplished in my field, taught many successful courses, and become a father of a beautiful girl and the husband of a beautiful wife, living in Singapore teaching philosophy.

I had not planned for any of these dreams to come true. I had joined a Ph.D. program mainly on the advice of a great teacher of mine who would later become a co-author of some of my books, David Levine. He recommended that I study with the two most renowned psychoanalytic political philosophers of our time: C. Fred Alford and James M. Glass. They both happened to be at the University of Maryland, College Park. I had never even been to Maryland but I applied there and was accepted and even given a fellowship. I wanted only to learn more; the degree meant little to me.

As time passed, I ended up working as a Teaching Assistant and teaching undergraduate students. I was terrified at first and didn't think I could do it. What if I had a gap in my knowledge? What if I misled students or taught them incorrectly? In spite of these fears, I found that I loved this work and was good at it. It was not altogether unlike creative writing: I found that I was capable of being fully present with students. In a discussion, I didn't fear silence and was able to respond to students so that they could lead the way in developing their own understanding.

In more formal settings, I was able to give whole lectures spontaneously, off the top of my head, without slideshows or pages of notes. Lecturing while in the moment proved to be a totally different experience for me than what my peers experienced. They and their students got bored because they were constantly removed from the moment, from the present, and returned to a pre-planned, forced schedule of thoughts, dictated by a book chapter, some notecards, or a slide-deck.

I didn't know I wanted to become a teacher until I already had become one. I had followed one intuition toward the good and it had led me to another good. I was free to pick up this other good and to pursue it and I was even free to be good at it, if I followed my own natural talents and tendencies with patience. This was the meaning of "I can do anything."

I had another tattoo around this time which read somewhat differently. I had been studying and writing about absurdism and had struggled, in my own life, with feelings of absurdity, angst, exploitation, and unfreedom. My job was not ideal. Yes, I could teach and write, but my work environment was poor, the pay was poor, and there were regular abuses that left me feeling beaten up almost every day.

In spite of (or because of) (or both) these circumstances, I was as productive as ever. I had learned that my own brokenness did not have to be perceived as a block to my happiness or creativity. The more I grew comfortable with this intuition, the more discoveries I made and insights had into psychoanalysis and philosophy, the more I was able to write creative and penetrating works.

Because I was reading a lot in French at the time, I got a tattoo in French that said "Let it break," with a hint of "Let itself [yourself] be broken." It reminded me that being broken was not a dead end, nor was it a permanent state. In being broken, one could find truths that were not palatable to those busy holding themselves together, optimizing themselves, all the time.

This was, for me, a very quick summary of my rejection of the hundreds of self-help books, seminars, and teachings I had read in my life. None taught that it was okay to break. None taught that it was okay to break from desire; rather they taught that we had to harness desire and pursue it to achieve gain. Here I was, broken, and yet surrounded by abundance.

Perhaps the most famous Daoist teaching of Chuang-Tzu is the parable known as "The Useless Tree." Let me relate it here in its entirety.

> Hui Tzu said to Chuang: I have a big tree, the kind they call a "stink tree." The Trunk is so distorted, so full of knots, no one can get a straight plank out of it. The branches are so crooked you cannot cut them up in any way that makes sense. There it stands beside the road. No carpenter will even look at it. Such is your teaching – big and useless. Chuang Tzu replied: Have you ever watched the wildcat crouching, watching his prey – This way it leaps, and that way, high and low, and at last, lands in the trap. But have you seen the yak? Great as a thundercloud he stands in his might. Big? Sure, he can't catch mice! So for your big tree. No use? Then plant it in the wasteland in emptiness. Walk idly around, rest under its shadow; no axe or bill prepares its end. No one will ever cut it down. Useless? You should worry![8]

The tree is broken. It is so broken that no one will ever break it. In this way, we come to know that even our most serious brokenness won't kill us. It is survivable. Even when things fall apart, as they do, all is not lost. Even when all seems lost, something will come next. The crooked tree provides shade and is even a thing of unique beauty, in its own way. When we reflect on this we come to feel that our selves and our souls have been through a lot. Pain, suffering, tears, gashes, rips, breaks, agonies, along with paradoxes, confusions, and times of loss and strife, along with victories and moments of rapture have all contributed to our shape. No wonder we are gnarled and full of knots. It couldn't be any other way.

Notes

1 The reader may wish to cross-reference the account of being 'enlightened and/or depressed,' in Chapter 5.
2 M.H. Bowker, "Seven Postmodern Problems in No Particular Hierarchical Occidental Phallological Order," *Superficial Flesh* 5, no. 1 (2010): 64–65.
3 Friedrich Nietzsche, *Beyond Good and Evil: Prelude to a Philosophy of the Future*, trans. H. Zimmern (Edinburgh: T.N. Foulis, 1909), 24.
4 Thomas Merton, *The Climate of Monastic Prayer* (Kalamazoo, MI: Cistercian Publications, 1969), quoted in Thomas Merton, *Dialogues with Silence: Prayers and Drawings*, eds. Jonathan Montaldo (San Francisco: Harper San Francisco, 2001), xiii.
5 Winnicott, *The Maturational Processes and the Facilitating Environment* (New York: International Universities Press, 1965), 170.
6 Winnicott, *The Maturational Processes and the Facilitating Environment* (New York: International Universities Press, 1965), 372.
7 Adam Phillips, *Side Effects* (New York: Harper Perennial, 2007), 75.
8 Thomas Merton, *The Way of Chuang Tzu* (New York: New Directions, 1965), 35.

15 Bravery and *Working Through* Subjectivity in Psychoanalysis

I have suffered from mental illness for most of my life. I have been fortunate that, in large part, I have succeeded in pursuing my work (as a professor and writer) and my relationships (my lovely family) over and against what has been an ever-changing yet ever-present struggle.

I have been in psychoanalysis or psychotherapy for over 15 years, with temporary periods of counseling reaching back even further, and have been medicated in some way or other for over ten years.

My family has a history of mental illness that runs pretty deep. Either as a cause of effect of this, or both, growing up in my childhood home was an experience of conflict, trauma, and confusion for me, and, likely, for the other members of my family as well.

In this chapter, I present a highly selective compilation of responses (having attempted to weed out the banal and the repetitive) to my 12-year-long psychoanalytic treatment and my psychoanalyst's (rather minimalistic) behavior, prompting, and questioning during that period. (The "you" in the notes is always my psychoanalyst.) Everything in italics in this chapter was once a note, typed or hand-written, jotted down to help me do some honest critical thinking about my psychotherapy and about my progress.

I believe that, relatively recently, I found some answers to the very difficult questions and dilemmas raised here. And I believe I arrived at some resolution of these problems by way of the process of "brave" self-analysis and critical thinking.

Beyond any form of psychoanalytic study or psychotherapeutic treatment, developing my capacity for genuinely critical thought has been my savior. It runs counter to a great deal of spiritual self-help that teaches us either to disparage our thoughts as illusions of our destructive egos or to ignore our thoughts as mere distractions. On the contrary, it has only been through a method of critical thinking that I have been able to plumb the depths of my soul, to create from a place of true authenticity, and to center myself in my true being.

In any case, I hope you will find something of interest in what follows. I have tried to group the questions and notes by subject, but have probably only succeeded in doing so to a certain degree. What follows, then, are compilations

DOI: 10.4324/9781003626398-18

of somewhat raw notes from over a decade's worth of psychoanalytic treatment and self-reflection.

What Kind of Therapy Is This?

In the early stages of treatment, I felt confused about what kind of therapy I was doing. There are, of course, many different kinds of therapy. One kind is where the therapist is more of a life-coach who helps the patient by commenting on events and patterns happening in the patient's life, making suggestions, and offering ideas as to how to think differently. That was not the kind of therapy I was in.

There is another, more traditional, form of psychoanalysis in which the analyst is much less active. Here, the idea is that the patient and analyst mainly struggle through *the transference*, which means, basically, the patient's transferring of attributes, attitudes, and emotions onto the analyst that belong to parts of the self or others in his, her, or their life. This re-encountering in analysis permits a more contained re-experiencing of complex, early, and often traumatic dilemmas. This re-experiencing allows the patient to feel and view the related emotions more consciously and even, ideally, to put them where they actually belong.

On the subject of the transference and traumatic re-experiencing, in the context of a state of confusion about where I was and what I was doing, I wrote the following.

Sometimes, depending upon the nature of the disorder, I know that patients have to suffer excruciatingly in therapy, have to have a sort of breakdown in order to have a breakthrough. I am not sure if I am one of those cases. Your prodding to be "more emotional" sometimes feels like that is what you are hinting at, and yet, from what I know, the re-experiencing stage is often discussed in the context of a breakdown into psychosis for psychotic or borderline individuals. I am not sure if these categories apply to me, and it seems crazy to aim for a breakdown, so I don't know what I am aiming for.

I don't know what my goals are, what the process entails, what I am trying to do, what constitutes progress, what criteria exist for completing this process, how to know if I have succeeded, how to define the nature of the task, and how to articulate (if it can be articulated) what it is that I need or need to do.

Is it necessary for me to re-experience something here? Your inevitable failures as an analyst will not be the same as the big failures that got me here: Yours are more normal, perhaps more understandable, or, at any rate, I am more willing to forgive you and to understand, since you are not playing the part of my parent and I know that.

You seem willing and able to mend your errors or to try to, whereas this was not ever imaginable in my early life: My mother, for example, never apologized for a single thing in her life, never admitted she was wrong or made a mistake.

If I dared to point out a mistake to her, I was given a silent stare that meant: "I know best, I know all, and I am silently interpreting what you are doing now because one day you will see how foolish you are for saying what you are saying. By this silence, you now already ought to feel ashamed for feeling what you are feeling because you must and will agree with me that I am correct, that I know best and that whatever you think against me or against what has happened only actually reveals your stupidity and childishness and badness."

There are a lot of angles to consider here, but before we go into them all, I should say that I understand that this, itself, is part of my issue, itself a part of the analytic situation for me. I get that this is also a pattern in my relationships: confusion or frustration in which I do not know what I need or how to get it, or when the other party is fulfilling my needs and when the other party is failing. I also feel I am not permitted to just break things off if they are not working, since, frankly, I feel confused about whether things are working or not.

What Makes Me Crazy

In the following note, I am really struggling to figure out what my analyst wants from me. In some ways, this question is wrong-headed, because I should be more focused on what *I* need. But it is an understandable complication in analysis because you have, on one side, a very confused and upset patient, and, on the other, a doctor who seems to hold, who one imagines to hold, some answers. My impatience with the process and my desire for answers is highlighted here. Also apparent is my working through, with the imaginary analyst, a terrible dilemma I experienced in childhood. The analytic situation is repeating it and, in this sense, is doing what analysis is supposed to do, no matter how painful it is.

I am feeling really exasperated with all of this. Things are not happening fast enough. I am trying and trying and I feel like all you are doing is sitting there "being patient." I don't feel that you have a sense of urgency here, as my life is slipping away, day by day, hour by hour, week by week. I ask and ask for more help, for guidance, for opportunities to make changes or to gain insight. Yet I feel like I am refused, or given an answer that is unhelpful, given in a tone of sort of flat, calm, moderateness.

At the same time, you are asking me, in a way that I have already explained to be unhelpful for me, unsuited to my needs, to feel certain emotions. You have asked me try to feel certain things in your presence but have been unclear about what this means or how to do so. This makes me believe that you are saying I should be able to guess or intuit how to feel and how to be. How else can I think if you refuse to explain these things or offer me any alternative ways of approaching them?

Basically, I feel you are being intransigent. But then that leaves me to wonder if you are being intransigent just because it is your way or because there is something essential in what you are being intransigent about. If I have trouble connecting with an emotion you think I should feel, or if I have trouble connecting with any emotion at all when relating a story or event, I end up with the sensation of just beating my head up against a wall.

Sometimes I feel that in this analysis I am in a sort of cult, that there is a very vague demand and all my time I have to spend trying to guess what it is. This generates a sort of weird compliance and great expectations and confusion and hope when really it is actually a form of cruelty.

Here I am trying to guess at what "the guru" is saying in his confusing mystical speech, even though I feel I have no way of understanding what it really means or of giving you what you want – and I realize of course that this, itself, is pathological, that I should not being trying to give you what you want in my analysis, but rather I should be trying to do what works for me and get what I need.

In any case, all the time I spend trying to figure things out feels as if it is taking me further away from my real needs and my real life. But, by not being clear or by not clearly changing when I raise complaints, you effectively keep insisting upon your method. And in your method, it is not clear to me what I have to do or what the problem is or what exact steps I need to take to feel better.

It is like the way you keep bringing up that time when I asked if it was okay that I sort of hurled my heavy winter coat on one side of the couch. You made a big thing of this and used it as a metaphor for me asking if I was "allowed to be at home" here, in the room, with you. I understand the importance of the metaphor, but it was a humiliating moment for me and yet you keep returning to it. You know that I cried eventually as we sat with that question in the air. But then nothing happened. I had to pick myself up all by myself and pull myself together all by myself and now you just pick at the scab. And you bring it up and leave me alone in my experience of that vulnerability right at those moments when you are refusing to share with me anything of my emotional experience. It feels like you want to just provoke me into feeling pain or humiliating and then leave me to twitch and crumble alone. I know that all of these aspersions about you could be read as part of the transference. But that knowledge doesn't help me get through the reality of what you are doing and the reality of what was done to me when I was a child.

It feels cruel to be asked to re-experience emotional experiences by another person who refuses to share them with you, by a person who only asks that you have them in his presence, at his demand, but to have them alone, while he sits comfortably in a leather chair and takes notes and feels or believes or "knows" without a doubt that he is right to have demanded this of you.

It reminds me of the time when I was a very young child [age 4] and my mother asked me to spell "quiet" but wouldn't give me any clues and, in spite of my proficiency at spelling, I couldn't guess it and I begged for help. Absolutely begged for help. And she refused even after I had a sort of breakdown, a total loss of control, a complete tantrum.

To be put in that position by my mother, was and, by you, is perverse, terrible, humiliating. It feels like a repetition of the childhood situation in which the cold or indifferent glance of the parent to the child's panic and fear and sadness and crisis stifles the child's emotions: because the child needs but lacks a mirror. Isn't it the same when you act cold and clinical while asking me to be emotional or excited or "alive"? This is not you being a mirror or a facilitator. In fact, it is you putting me in an impossible position that I can't get out of: I can't feel things in that situation, but I also am told that I must feel things to get out of that situation.

This whole situation I find terribly humiliating, because it feels like capitulation, to you, to your demands, and even if capitulation might "cure" one part of me (which I doubt), it would make another part of me sick, like the dream of the monastery, where the cure of going into a monastery and giving up all I love is worse than the disease.

I sometimes feel that I cannot and will never give you what you want in this way, and if I did, it would be an utter defeat and I don't know how I would be able to face myself again.

If I did somehow figure out what you wanted from me in here, what experience or emotion you needed for me to have, then gave it, did it, performed it, surrendered to it . . . that would be in some sense the ultimate humiliation, the ultimate disgusting shameful display. That would be me allowing myself to be "mind-fucked" by you, to be violated, to be turned inside out at your behest. I cannot and will not do that. So, if that is still something you think is necessary for me, then I have to leave and find a new analyst where this dynamic can be worked out in some other way, since I think we are at a real impasse.

What (I Think) I Need and Don't Need

One of the most crucial themes in my analysis was "getting something I need." I think, after years of reflection, that there was something I missed as a child and I never got what I needed. In analysis, faced with what seemed to be a tantalizing opportunity to get the thing I always needed, I was full of angst and fear.

I NEED for you to tell me what I NEED to do in order to get what I NEED from you.

That is the key sentence for the moment.

And you won't tell me, I suspect, or you will say something, but won't explain it adequately, so even this need will be frustrated: My need to know what I need to do to get what is needed will be frustrated.

Thus, the need to do the thing that is needed is also frustrated and the need at the bottom of it all to get the thing that is desperately needed is frustrated but is so buried beneath other frustrations that I never seem to get to feel that frustration, which is also something I need to do, because at the moment I don't even know what that thing is that I want to get: Is it love, is it acceptance, is it permission to be myself, is it protection and safety?

How can I know what it is if I can't even get to the point of feeling that I can't get it because there are other things I can't get that prevent me from getting to that point that are also denied or unavailable?

You said I seemed more "alive" today and I think that may be true. I think that experience is what I need. I said it is "because I am desperate" and that is true, too. What I felt and knew and maybe should reflect on is the fact that it also felt like violence, as if my aliveness were taking liberties with someone else, like a kind of recklessness, perhaps a recklessness at being willing to use and push and question and challenge and say things directly and possibly hurt the feelings of someone else, even or especially you, someone whom I care about and someone who is entrusted to care about me.

What I don't need is when you say things like you have "enjoyed my visits" for these years while I have been very often in great pain and suffering, losing my life, watching and feeling my soul drain out of me agonizingly in anxiety and pain and shame and fear. The idea that you have been "enjoying" watching me do this and in some sense facilitating this slow torture is very hard to handle. So much that when I dare to question the torture I feel you breaking things off with me. The whole thing then makes me feel sick and angry.

This business about enjoyment is a pattern. People have "enjoyed" me even when I was miserable. My parents enjoyed me performing functionally even when I was terribly upset and terrified for much of my childhood. I wonder, though, how someone can enjoy someone when that person is so unhappy, is not enjoying themselves? Do you have to be disconnected from their emotional centers? Is that enjoyment not like exploitation of a sort, where the real person is not seen or dealt with, only the parts that are enjoyable are used and the rest is cut out, left off, pushed away, swept under the rug? This, of course, only increases my sense of misery and unhappiness, misrecognition, and disconfirmation, and a kind of enforcement of a false self in the relationship in which only the "enjoyable" self is being related to, only the "enjoyable" self is welcome.

"False Self" Reflections

These reflections led me to think more about the "false self" front I erected in childhood and the possibility that it had remained with me into adult life. As discussed above in Chapter 4, the false self is created as a way to satisfy others, by seeming functional, content, capable, or even happy. This note continued from the last, on the subject of being "enjoyable" to visit with.

I have learned, sometimes consciously and sometimes unconsciously, to be an enjoyable (false) self, to deliver painful and sad news with a smile or a joke, to be aware of what the other person wants to hear so that I can manage my impression and not be too unenjoyable. This includes being a sensitive relationship-partner.

Thus, in this context and in this sense, I exploit myself: I make myself into a false enjoyable self and reap certain rewards of this: esteem, friendship, decent relations with people, colleagues, you.

It earns one a certain kind of respect, even love – but it isn't true love – or rather this is where I am confused – it is the only love I have ever known, excepting perhaps with my own family. Actually, it is scary for me to call it "false" love, because it is the only kind I think I had growing up.

Last time, an emotion landed for me when I found myself asking what was so wrong with me that my parents behaved the way that they did. I felt and noticed a difficulty in being without some "false self" props. Anxiety, itself, felt like a tool to keep a false self intact. I felt as if I was in a predicament where, if I let anxiety go and just was, I would fall apart, or do something terrible, or be something terrible, grotesque, or unlovable.

Sometimes, the more I sit and think and feel deeply, I think that "left to my own devices" I am disgusting. Thus, the split between the true and false self is maintained for me through anxiety: Anxiety keeps the true self from appearing without scrutiny and censorship and sometimes ironic, instantaneous, self-reflective commentary. The false self is where my value is stored, hence my difficulty enjoying things where my earned, conditional self-regard is harder to find: in "just being," on vacation, on my birthday, when I am just a person, not a special, accomplished person.

In Response to a Query About Anger

My analyst asked me to think about something that made me angry and implied that I had difficulty with the emotion of anger. I couldn't think of anything in the moment. This is what I thought of later.

My father used to tell a story about a young man who goes to Paris to paint but needs help at first from his parents to support his dreams, fails to make it on his own, and eventually writes a one-word telegram home because it is all he can afford. The telegram says: "Starving." The two-word reply from home, at least somewhat contrary to what we might expect, and a glorious reply in my father's eyes, which he was always elated to tell, so elated that he could almost not wait to get to the punchline, was: "So starve."

It is worth noting that my father used to tell me this story around the time that I went to Paris to study. My father did not discriminate greatly between my desire to pursue academics (which I did ultimately pursue) and the desire of the artist in the story to pursue painting. In fact, he used to sneer at professors as "academicians," which always had a rather pernicious, nasal tone about it.

So, what is so cruel about this story? I suppose one cruelty was the sheer number of times I heard it, as if it were meant for me. There is also the inherent cruelty of the parents' response to the child's plea for help, a kind of tough love unto death. For me, I always felt that there was another message in the story, aimed at me, which was: "You will fail, unless . . ." And the "unless" here would have to be some kind of fairly strict pragmatism as regards career and work. And this message, in turns, meant to me: "You are not good enough to have a great dream or to succeed in a way that is meaningful for you. Instead, you will fail and seek dependency, until you are forced by necessity to get a more secure job."

This is only one of many stories and interactions I had with my parents throughout my life that seemed aimed at convincing me that I was not good enough to aim for anything more than survival, that, even worse, wishing for more was shameful and childish. What awaited adults who were not childish was a thankless and sorrowful life of work, saving, boredom, and ultimately sacrificing oneself to one's own children who would require financial support. It was a pretty bleak outlook, but it was his way of trying to protect me from ruin.

Why teach a child that he is nothing special, that dreaming equals starving, that he will always fail, all for his own good? I think back to how many times my father invoked Maslow's hierarchy, which he did not fully understand, to convey the need for securing survival-basics first and everything else later. I think perhaps I am angry that I did not have parents who encouraged me to dream, who could have even helped me dream, and who would have helped me dream dreams that I would be fulfilled in a meaningful way, actualized my potential, and found happiness. Instead, really out of fear, the lesson of my parents was the lesson of how not to dream, how to reject dreamers and dreaming.

I think I have, in spite of all of this, dreamed. And I have dreamed even though dreaming has brought me a fair share of guilt and anxiety.

Last night I cried about the way that people and situations in my life (including therapy at this moment) made it so difficult to like (much less love) life, made it impossible to enjoy or look forward to things, made it feel like a prison camp, as if the only way out would be death, and even death would involve disgrace, so really there is no way out, only suffering.

In Response to a Query about a Childhood Theme

My analyst asked me to think about a theme of my childhood and I came up with something like *self-inflicted suffering*. Here is what I wrote.

I should say that I think my mother wanted me to suffer in order to ensure that I wouldn't be "soft." And I obliged, in my own strange way. At age 8, I had taken to beating myself up and coming home with bruises and cuts in an attempt to win the curious combination of sympathy and approval I longed for.

Sneaking across the driveway of our house in a Chicago suburb, I ducked underneath the kitchen window and crawled into the side yard where patches of hard ice gathered underneath the icicles on the small porch. I broke off clumps of ice and smashed myself in the head with them, then buried my face in an embankment until it was covered with snow. I would enter the house quietly and stoically. To my chagrin, my mother never asked what happened, never worried, never held me. I repeated the procedure for several days until finally I announced that I was being attacked by the local bully, Chris Harrison. My mother noted the name. Chris Harrison did bully us younger kids, but never at the perfect time when our suffering could be seen.

Since I felt denied what I desired, I continued to invent ways of hurting myself, including unnecessary spills out of a large apple tree in the back yard, innumerable tumbles off of the bike I taught myself to ride, and other skinned-knee accidents. Once, I even stabbed myself in the thigh with a pencil in school. I thought I was building quite a case for victimization, but one day, my mother sat me down and calmly told me that she had investigated my earlier accusations by visiting the Harrison home. Chris' mother apparently informed mine that Chris had been out of school with mono for several of the days in question, and thus, he could not have injured me as I had said. I had lied. And, in a humiliating ritual, I was forced to remove my pants and was spanked naked by my mother, then grounded as punishment.

By age 9, I was pulling out my hair in small clumps and biting my fingernails halfway to the cuticle. I still cannot eat most processed ham because our sickly neurotic cat, Lila, was, for her own reasons, also destroying herself. Lila was gnawing off all of the hair off of her own left side, leaving only a raw, pink, boney flank of cat flesh that looked eerily similar to the hairless pink scalp gradually making itself visible all over my own head. This pink flesh is all I can see when I look at my mother's favored brand of lunch meat.

By the time I was 10 we had moved to another suburb, this time outside of Dallas, and victimization had become an integral part of my personality, so when my friends and I would inevitably run into trouble with the two or three older kids on our block and get into a fight, I relished it. With a degree of regularity and predictability, the older kids, large football players at the local junior high, would engage themselves in our play, whatever it was: street soccer, football, frisbee. As the game went on, our interactions would become increasingly unruly, the pushes and bumps increasingly more illegal, until, in a kind of eruption of violence, the older kids would unleash fists, elbows, and chokeholds on us.

I secretly loved these moments. As an athletic kid, I was not unable to mount a decent defense, not one good enough to defeat a group of larger and stronger kids, but all that was not important. What was important was getting struck across the jaw by someone and hearing your ears ring like a bell. Or being punched in the stomach and having the wind knocked out of you, with its attendant feelings of nausea and desperation. Or being choked from behind and lifted off of your feet until you flail to regain control of your breath. I was never badly hurt, and was never really worried about being hurt in these fights or any others. In fact, being hurt was the goal. If I had defeated my opponent, the beating would not have served its purpose, because in the act of fighting I would have given the bigger kid a right to be the victim. As it was, it was pure innocent victimization, and it was glorious.

As you might expect, I used to fantasize about my parents beating me, but they did not. Except for a couple of spankings which were more violent psychologically than physically, my parents never laid a hand on me. Indeed, I think a smack might have been some kind of intimate contact in an otherwise chilly, dark home. Even at 6, I had found ways to make suffering count as contact, as I began to develop chest pains and difficulty breathing in my First Grade classroom. After a few weeks of being told it was nothing, my parents noticed bruises in a line across my sternum and asked me where they came from. Ms. Helie's preferred method for quieting children down, it turned out, was to ask them to put their heads on their desks. Since I innocently assumed that this directive was a form of punishment, it did not occur to me to slide my chair out and lie comfortably on the desk, as all the other children did. Thus, sitting flush with the small desk, I attempted each day to press my forehead down to the table top, creating an agonizing pressure as the edge of the desktop pushed into my chest and abdomen. But I was glad and grateful each day when Ms. Helie lovingly ended the punishment, which must have lasted 4 or 5 minutes but which seemed to last hours, for it meant that all was forgiven.

Everything considered, my history could have been much, much worse. I could have been sexually abused or physically tortured by my parents. I was not. That fact is a source of something like shame for me, because I FELT *as if I had been abused and tortured. And I manifested that abuse and torture in my life even if I had to make it happen myself. The terms "psychological abuse" and "emotional neglect" did not do justice to the agony I felt as a child. Rather, I lived in a world where I was described as the obedient child one moment, and as a "rotten," "horrible" child the next. If I had ever done anything aggressive, like screamed, about this or about the pain I felt inside, I think the house would have fallen apart, something would have cracked, perhaps my parents would have divorced, or someone would have died from the strain.*

Fortunately, I was somehow able to cordon off a tiny part of my self that could not be touched by all the fear, shame, and negative attributions surrounding me. It was the part of me that knew I was innocent, even though I had been guilty of effectively lying about victimization in order to get treated as an innocent. If I had analyzed this part of myself, or even known it was there as a younger man, I fear it might have disappeared. I think perhaps it had to be and still has to be my secret in order for me to remain vital.

I think about this theme, now, in this way: I am willing to go through all of this – pain, misery, self-inflicted suffering, repetition of traumatic patterns and agonizing feelings in the transference, etc. – but only if it is going to get me somewhere. Then again, I worry: Isn't the idea that I have to go through all of this agony with someone, just to get somewhere (i.e., to get something from them) actually part of my particular pattern? That is, does this process repeat and reaffirm all of the things that I thought I was trying to break away from? That includes the idea that I have to suffer inordinately in order to receive a modicum of care that, then, is spoiled by having had to suffer disproportionately, so it can't even be enjoyed, having to suffer the humiliation of my resistance in the end when it is revealed that the pain I was suffering was necessary but I protested it as if it were not necessary or excessive? Having to accept that the same person who was harming me was harming me "for my own good," making me really split, divided, confused about how to feel about the cruel, caring, hurtful, depriving, yet well-intended person?

I think I am just confused about whether this is working through trauma or whether it is re-traumatization, making things worse, digging in deeper. How can I know?

Seeking and Avoiding Traumatic Repetition

Finally, after years of work, reflection, and critical self-analysis, I think I started to make some headway in my analysis. This coincided with a feeling of being more of an agent, more of a subject, more of a responsible party, and less of a victim. Coming to this subjective state with respect to analysis is scary, because if one feels one has made a misstep, it can all fall apart. But here are some of my later thoughts.

I know I have a right not to have my relationships be like this, not to be frustrating, tormenting, and persecutory. I can choose to give up the persecution, but only in tandem with giving up false hope. And I see that, in some way, I have needed to hold on to the false hope as well as the experience of persecution until now. And this has left me feeling very powerless and hopeless. But now I feel that I have a bit of power and a bit of hope because I feel that I can give those up. Until now I didn't really see that I needed both or that the two were connected.

Of course, giving these up means realizing that the false hope was once a true hope, a hope that wasn't fulfilled yet should have been fulfilled, and therefore having the feelings of anger and sadness that go along with recognizing that fact. It means putting the hope in its proper place, which is really in the past but also in my present insofar as I have been holding onto it, and it means no longer trying to recapture it now, but dealing with the fact that it is gone, that it never was, and that it should have been, and that this has been a real source of suffering for me.

I think it been very hard for me even to articulate what this hope was or is, but over the past few weeks I have been hoping all the time that instead of the relationship we have, for instance, or even the relationship I have with others or with work or with the world, I could have a relationship with a nurturing parent, in ways that exceed what I think you can and should do, in ways that realistically I don't expect or even want, but this made it very hard for me to see what I did truly want and, subsequently, to 'realize what I have now realized, which is that what I wanted was once theoretically possible but then soon after impossible and now, especially since my parents are dead, truly impossible.

I feel that I know now more about what I want out of analysis, and not only that, but how I want it to proceed, what I want and need are more available to me because they are more realistic, they are more clear because they are not so deeply confused with what I once wanted and failed to find. This is hard, and I still have to work through all of the feelings associated with that early loss, that failure to find, but that I can see as one of my goals, and it doesn't require that I be in a sick or twisted frustration and torment-filled relationship with my analyst.

Part of asserting this right is giving up on the expectation of impossible emotional perfection, because it is this expectation that, when it is failed or missed, creates the feeling of persecution. The feeling of persecution is proportional to the degree of impossible perfection that is unreasonably expected. NOT *to bring that expectation, along with the expectation of frustration and failure, into analysis is to find the possibility of a more limited and reasonable sort of relationship that actually serves my needs, needs that can be met or at least potentially can be met, rather than serving a more unconscious need to demand perfect care that is unreasonable and, at the same time, that serves my need to re-experience the agony and suffering associated with this need being unmet.*

Of course, part of this is realizing that I might not need to have been doing all of this if my parents had given me what I needed when I needed it: Those needs were unmet and really now can never be fully met since they are in the past. Feeling all that pain and anger now at those people who failed in the past will help me from re-experiencing in unwanted ways the same pain in new situations when new people really aren't the ones to blame (at least not on the exact same terms).

This involves the idea that I can assert myself in therapy and try to trust my own feelings and instincts about what kind of relationship I really want it to be, and what I want to get out of it. I can make "terms" of my own if I want, and those terms can be possible and not impossible, and they can be met. This more reasonable meeting of needs is a better pattern than going around trying both to find and to fail to find someone who will meet the needs of an infant like a mother who already did not meet them and who is now dead.

This is my desire: to have you be a loving parent. Yet this desire is impossible and even though it is impossible it is also *my desire to (re)create this same situation where you fail to be my loving parent, which is frustrating, enraging, horrible. Now that I am re-experiencing all of that, extremely powerfully, from this experience and this knowledge I can conclude that I will never again find the loving parent that I never had, and that it is crazy of me to seek it in people who cannot possibly serve that function for me, and that it is also crazy to (unconsciously) seek the experience of disappointment and frustration and rage that comes from re-experiencing this failure in others, since my desire to re-experience even these awful emotions is in some sense my attempt to hang on to my mother, or my fantasies about her, or some crazy hope that maybe the next time she (or the person or group representing her at that moment) will actually come out perfect and she will give me everything I need.*

She will never be there, she will never give me what I need. Even now when I think of her and about family, it still fills me with fear. I always thought this fear was normal, that everyone felt afraid of their families, of going home, of being at home. I am still working through all of these feelings but I have felt hatred and resentment and I have accused both mother and father of terrible things and I feel okay about those accusations, and I have felt sorry for myself, and sad and incredibly angry that I had to suffer this and that the effects of this are still with me, consistently, continually depriving me of life and joy and happiness. I am "sick" of it, really – I am sick with it all, I am disgusted by it, disgusted by what passed for a family and for love, which was really a terrible deprivation, control rather than care, a business arrangement and social engineering project rather than warmth or love.

That said, I would say my more mature goals in therapy are these:

1. *To try to process the feelings associated with giving up the expectation of perfection and seeing the feelings of persecution as attached to this expectation, and to an unconscious desire to keep experiencing frustration, and to some false hope that maybe this time the persecution will turn into relief and satisfaction, and as a way to defend against the settling for lesser satisfactions that I should be able to settle for now but that I should not have had to settle for as a child, and therefore to defend against feelings of anger and sadness associated with the fact that I had to settle when I shouldn't have had to settle.*
2. *To receive helpful support and advice about how I can redefine my goals in therapy and in life so that I am not looking for something that cannot be provided, and to talk about times and situations where I may be still seeking that which I do not really want to seek.*
3. *To learn and to have you support and build up my confidence and self-esteem. In part, this includes some greater sensitivity on your part about saying things that feel to me like criticisms of my ability to feel. I would rather the environment support and recognize that I am trying very hard, and to be just a little more positive rather than only pointing out my failures, which I admit to having. This is important because if I am going to assert myself I need to overcome deep-seated feelings of worthlessness and shame and self-hatred and feel, instead, that I can trust myself and my instincts and that they won't always lead me to disaster.*

Maybe the answer to all of this, the upshot, is maybe it doesn't have to be like this: that even therapy doesn't have to be like this. Maybe I have the power to stop creating and participating in situations and experiences like this if I don't want to. To stop setting them up with certain expectations and other dynamics that create this thing for me. That would mean I could make the therapy whatever I want it to be, and that would mean I wouldn't be imprisoned in it. I could choose to use it as I see fit and when I feel my aims are met or even if I feel that they can't be met I could leave and not have to feel guilt and shame about that.

That would be freedom. I have never known this kind of freedom. It is hard for me to imagine, and I think I still have to work through some of the blockades that I throw up at times when I contemplate or am presented with the possibility of this freedom. But that, at least, is something that I can see coming out of this: that I don't have to be trapped like this. If I find myself in a frustrating or anxiety-provoking situation I can address it on its own terms, and I can reflect upon what I have brought to the table that has given it this meaning as well, and I can reflect on and reassess my expectations and I can assert my power to not be in that situation any more, either by leaving it or by redefining the dynamic, re-establishing what works for me or the ground-rules that I need. As long as those can be respected, I can continue to have a relationship that is good for me without the accompanying fear and frustration.

Conclusion

Thinking, Happiness, and the Problem with Eckhart Tolle

"All problems are illusions of the mind."

– Eckhart Tolle

Since the notes in the previous chapter were written, I have finished with my 12-year analysis and now see a therapist who is less strictly analytic, more of a psycho-dynamically oriented counselor. Looking back, it was a great deal of work. Some people who knew I was working this hard in psychoanalysis felt it was a waste of time and effort, as I sometimes felt, myself. They were exasperated at the idea of spending 12 years *working through* issues such as these. But, for me, and perhaps just for me and not for everyone, it was a way to think, un-think, and re-think my position in life, my subjectivity.

In my view, Eckhart Tolle, famed spiritual leader, is wrong. The phrase above, that "all problems are illusions of the mind," in the context of his book, *The Power of Now*, is taken to mean that thinking is always or primarily negative, that thinking cannot be a path to "presence." Tolle claims that thinking must subside for presence to arise.[1]

In my own experience, and in my work, study, and teaching, I have found thinking, particularly *honest, patient, and brave critical thinking*, to be absolutely necessary for my own subjective presence to find its place. This book has argued that the path to subjectivity lies in thinking and not in its avoidance. In this brief Conclusion, I just want to say a final word about the power of thinking, against one of its greatest critics.

In Tolle, we find an attack on thinking, as if thinking itself were responsible for "all problems," as if we should just stop thinking and then become happier. Thinking can, like all things, lead to both positive and negative outcomes, but there is a way to use thinking to find better, fuller states of being, to think oneself out of denial and repression, even to get to "the now." It is true that sometimes we can defend against feeling by thinking, intellectualizing, or rationalizing, but a truly self-honest, emotionally patient, and psychologically brave stance should help us see through these and related defenses.

DOI: 10.4324/9781003626398-19

Part of the problem with this debate is that people like Tolle seem to believe that being "present" in "the now" is always or primarily pleasant: In "the now," you automatically appreciate your surroundings, your body, and your aliveness and you say, "Oh how beautiful that I am alive and have a body," or you look at the sky or the tree and say again, "How lovely."

I would argue that this is naïve. Being truly present with oneself means sometimes being in a very unpleasant state: a state of illness, pain, boredom, desire, anxiety, terror, and obsession. Finding "the now," in other words, does not release us from the human condition, which is in many ways a tragic condition, in which we are in many ways stuck in our limited bodies, aware we are stuck in them, aware we are going to die soon and forever, living in a universe bigger than we can comprehend where our actions may be utterly meaningless, subject to attachments to and histories with others whom we did not get to choose, possessing minds and psyches that are not entirely under our control, feeling feelings and desires we often can't act on or even fully know.

To add to that, we each have some degree of personal pain: the pain we have suffered in our own lives, due to history or experience, psychological makeup, physical health or unhealth, scars and vulnerabilities, weaknesses, and so on. One's personal pain is also human pain in the sense that others, while not suffering exactly as one has suffered, can relate, and have suffered similar or worse or less terrible things all to varying degrees.

So being in "the now" also entails being in human pain. I don't think we have to relish our human pain, and there is nothing wrong with doing things that take our minds off of it for a while, but I do think we should accept that it is there, that it is real, that finding it is not some "illusion" or "error." Recognizing that there is such a thing as human pain, and that others have had it, and that it is real, can make one feel more grounded, more free, more human, and more alive.

I am not released from pain. I continue to feel human pain, as I have for most of my life. There are several ways one could explain this, either sympathetically (i.e., I have emotional sensitivity, an accurate perception of the human condition, an unwillingness to resort to the usual defense mechanisms) or unsympathetically (I have an anxiety disorder, I am "over-thinking," I had a troubled childhood, etc.), but these explanations don't really matter so long as human pain is not blamed on the individual who merely experiences it simply because he, she, or they experience it.

I have suggested here that there is nothing greater, nothing nobler than to undertake the work of radical, honest, patient, brave, critical thinking, regarding oneself and regarding the world one inhabits.

Thinking is the work. We ought not get rid of thinking any more than we ought to get rid of feeling. It is our daily bread.

And, although thinking can lead us in almost any direction, one of its by-products is a kind of contentment: the contentment we find when our critical thinking joins up with our emotional maturity and honestly, patiently, and bravely declares that we can, to a great degree, shape our experience of the world as subjects, as the authors of our lives.

Note

1 Eckhart Tolle, *The Power of Now: A Guide to Spiritual Enlightenment* (Novato, CA: New World Library, 2004), 64.

References

Alford, C. Fred. *Whistleblowers: Broken Lives and Organizational Power*. Ithaca, NY: Cornell University Press, 2001.

Bollas, Christopher. *The Shadow of the Object: Psychoanalysis of the Unthought Known*. New York: Columbia University Press, 1987, 277–83.

Bowker, Matthew H. "Activity, Speech, and Change: Progressive Politics and Regressive Fantasies." *Psychoanalysis, Culture & Society* 24, no. 2 (2019): 105–17.

Bowker, Matthew H. "Analytic and Political Neutrality: Change, Privilege, and Responsibility." *Free Associations* 71 (2018): 1–17.

Bowker, Matthew H. *Critical Thinking and the Subject of Inquiry: Capacities, Resilience, and Power*. Redwood City, CA: Bluemount, 2025.

Bowker, Matthew H. *Ideologies of Experience: Trauma, Failure, Deprivation, and the Abandonment of the Self*. New York and London: Routledge, 2016.

Bowker, Matthew H. *Misinterest: Essays, Pensées, and Dreams*. Santa Barbara, CA: Punctum Books, 2019.

Bowker, Matthew H. "Seven Postmodern Problems in No Particular Hierarchical Occidental Phallological Order." *Superficial Flesh* 5, no. 1 (2010): 64–65.

Bowker, Matthew H. "Teaching Students to Ask Questions Instead of Answering Them." *Thought and Action: The NEA Higher Education Journal* 26, no. 1 (2010): 127–34.

Bowker, Matthew H., and Amy Buzby, eds. *D.W. Winnicott and Political Theory: Recentering the Subject*. New York: Palgrave Macmillan, 2017.

Bowker, Matthew H., and K. Patrick Fazioli. "Rethinking Critical Thinking: A Relational and Practical Approach." *Pedagogy and the Human Sciences* 6, no. 1 (2016): 1–26.

Browning, Christopher R. *Ordinary Men: Reserve Police Battalion 101 and the Final Solution in Poland*. New York: HarperCollins, 1992.

Cleary, Thomas. *The Spirit of Tao*. Boston: Shambhala Publications, 1998, 73–74.

Fairbairn, W.R.D. "The Repression and the Return of Bad Objects." In *Psychoanalytic Studies of the Personality*, 59–81. London: Routledge & Kegan Paul, 1952.

Freud, Sigmund. *Beyond the Pleasure Principle*. Translated by James Strachey. New York: W.W. Norton & Company, 1961.

Lao Tzu. *Tao Te Ching*. Translated by John C.H. Wu. Boston: Shambhala Publications, 1989.

Levine, David P., and Matthew H. Bowker. *The Destroyed World and the Guilty Self: A Psychoanalytic Study of Culture and Politics*. London: Phoenix Publishing, 2019.

Marcuse, Herbert. "Repressive Tolerance." In *A Critique of Pure Tolerance*, edited by Robert Paul Wolff, Barrington Moore Jr., and Herbert Marcuse, 95–137. Boston: Beacon Press, 1969.

Merton, Thomas. *The Way of Chuang Tzu*. New York: New Directions, 1965, 35.

Milgram, Stanley. *Obedience to Authority: An Experimental View*. New York: Harper & Row, 1974.

Milne, A.A. *When We Were Very Young*. New York: Dutton, 1924.

Mitchell, Stephen, trans. *Tao Te Ching*. New York: Harper & Row, 1988, Chapter 17.

Phillips, Adam. *Side Effects*. New York: Harper Perennial, 2007, 75.

Robbins, Tom. *Jitterbug Perfume*. New York: Bantam Books, 1984.

Smail, David. *Illusion and Reality: The Meaning of Anxiety*. London: J.M. Dent & Sons, 1984.

Stevens, Wallace. "How to Live. What to Do." In *The Collected Poems of Wallace Stevens*, 125–26. New York: Vintage Books, 1990.

Tocqueville, Alexis de. *Democracy in America*. Translated by Harvey C. Mansfield and Delba Winthrop. Chicago: University of Chicago Press, 2000.

Tolle, Eckhart. *The Power of Now: A Guide to Spiritual Enlightenment*. Novato, CA: New World Library, 2004, 64.

Winnicott, D.W. "Ego Integration in Child Development." In *The Maturational Processes and the Facilitating Environment*, 56–63. New York: International Universities Press, 1965.

Winnicott, D.W. *Home is Where We Start From: Essays by a Psychoanalyst*. Edited by Clare Winnicott, Ray Shepherd, and Madeleine Davis. New York: W.W. Norton & Company, 1986.

Winnicott, D.W. *The Maturational Processes and the Facilitating Environment*. New York: International Universities Press, 1965.

Winnicott, D.W. *Playing and Reality*. London: Tavistock Publications, 1971.

Winnicott, D.W. "The Theory of the Parent-Infant Relationship." In *The Maturational Processes and the Facilitating Environment*, 37–55. New York: International Universities Press, 1965.

Index

For Product Safety Concerns and Information please contact our EU representative GPSR@taylorandfrancis.com
Taylor & Francis Verlag GmbH, Kaufingerstraße 24, 80331 München, Germany

www.ingramcontent.com/pod-product-compliance
Ingram Content Group UK Ltd.
Pitfield, Milton Keynes, MK11 3LW, UK
UKHW022016111225
465993UK00008B/664
* 9 7 8 1 0 4 1 0 4 0 0 9 5 *